Handbook of Leprosy

Handbook of Leprosy

W. H. Jopling FRCP (Lond), FRCP (Edin), DTM & H (Eng)

Formerly Consultant Leprologist, Hospital for Tropical Diseases, London, and Consultant in Tropical Dermatology, St John's Hospital for Diseases of the Skin, London.

A. C. McDougall MD (Edin), FRCP (Lond), MRCP (Edin)

Formerly Leprosy Specialist for the Ministry of Health, Lusaka, Zambia. Now Consultant in Clinical Investigation (Leprosy), British Leprosy Relief Association (LEPRA), Department of Dermatology, Slade Hospital, Headington, Oxford.

FOURTH EDITION

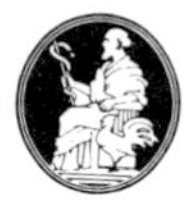

HEINEMANN PROFESSIONAL PUBLISHING

Heinemann Medical Books
An imprint of Heinemann Professional Publishing Ltd
Halley Court, Jordan Hill, Oxford OX2 8EJ

OXFORD LONDON MELBOURNE AUCKLAND

First published 1971
Second edition 1978
Third edition 1984
Fourth edition 1988

British Library Cataloguing in Publication Data

Jopling, W. H. (William Henry)
Handbook of leprosy. — 4th ed.
1. Man. Leprosy
I. Title II. McDougall, A. C.
616.9'98

ISBN 0–433–217569–9

Photoset and printed in Great Britain by
Redwood Burn Limited, Trowbridge, Wiltshire
and bound by Pegasus Bookbinding, Melksham, Wiltshire

Contents

Illustrations

COLOUR PLATES

TABLES

Preface to the First Edition

For a long time I have been impressed by the demand for information on leprosy from all sections of the medical and nursing professions, and I have attempted, in this Handbook, to give the basic facts about the disease and its management as clearly and conscisely as possible. During my visit to leprosy centres in Africa in 1968 I noted the responsible work undertaken by para-medical workers and their eagerness to do it well; I have particularly in mind the medical assistants in charge of rural clinics or travelling in Land-Rovers as members of mobile medical teams, and I hope that these workers and their counterparts in other developing regions will find in this volume the help they need.

As regards the medical profession, I hope that this Handbook will give the student and general practitioners a better understanding of leprosy, and will also have an appeal to the specialist on whom the diagnosis of the disease may fall, especially the dermatologist and the neurologist.

I would like to thank my son-in-law, Mr David Dartnall, for the drawings and diagrams, and I am grateful to Dr Colin McDougall and Dr Tin Shwe for helpful criticism and advice.

W. H. Jopling, 1971

Preface to the Fourth Edition

The fact that this *Handbook of Leprosy* now has two authors is indicative of the increasing scope of all aspects of the disease. We hope that the book will show that leprosy is not too complicated for all readers to understand, and that through the application of knowledge it will be controlled and eventually eradicated. In furtherance of this goal, it is important to have an informed medical profession, and we would urge those who train medical students in endemic countries to give to leprosy much more teaching time than is given at present in most medical colleges.

Valuable information is now being gained from reports of trials of multidrug therapy, confirming the acceptability of this line of chemotherapy as regards side-effects and administration during pregnancy. We anticipate a radical reduction in length of treatment of multibacillary leprosy, especially as trials have confirmed that chemotherapy can be stopped in spite of the presence of granular bacilli in smears or biopsies, and it is likely that follow-up studies will unravel the significance of small numbers of 'persisters' (living, drug-sensitive bacilli) which may be found at the time of stopping treatment. In view of the limited number of antileprosy drugs in current use, and the threat of increasing drug resistance posed by *M. leprae*, the search for new antileprosy drugs is of great importance. Hence, we welcome news from the WHO that trials in Côte d'Ivoire of two fluorinated quinolone derivatives, pefloxacin and ofloxacin, are producing promising results.

We endorse what was written in the preface to the first edition of this book about the important role of paramedicals (medical auxiliaries) in the control of this challenging disease, and we hope that those who have access to this edition will make use of the Glossary when they come across terms which are new to them.

(Throughout the book the patient and the leprologist/leprosy worker have been referred to as 'he', and it should be noted that this has been done for reasons of clarity and convenience only.)

Finally, we thank Dr Richard Barling of Heinemann Medical Books for his encouragement and cooperation in the production of this edition, and Miss Caroline Creed for all her help in the editing of our manuscript.

W. H. Jopling, A. C. McDougall, 1988

1 Definition, Epidemiology and World Distribution

DEFINITION

Leprosy (Hansen's disease (HD); Hanseniasis) is a chronic disease caused by *Mycobacterium leprae* (*M. leprae*), infectious in some cases, and affecting the peripheral nervous system, the skin, and certain other tissues.

EPIDEMIOLOGY

The rate at which leprosy spreads in a community depends on the proportion of susceptible persons in the population and the opportunities for contact with *M. leprae*. The view that adults are relatively insusceptible is supported by two observations: first, all attempts to infect volunteers have failed, and second, the incidence of conjugal leprosy (leprosy acquired from a marriage partner) is only about 5%. It would seem that children are more susceptible, for where children are at risk because of leprosy in the family, up to 60% develop the disease as children or young adults after an incubation period of 2–7 years (usually 3–5 years). Until recently it has been generally accepted that leprosy bacilli do not cross the placenta, but there are now grounds for believing that transplacental transmission of *M. leprae* may occur as a rare event,[1] thus accounting for a number of reports of clinical leprosy developing in infants. Reports of long incubation periods should be treated with caution as early physical signs may be unobtrusive. The mode of transmission is not yet known for certain, and three possible routes are under consideration, namely: the skin, the gastrointestinal tract and the respiratory tract (Fig. 1.1).

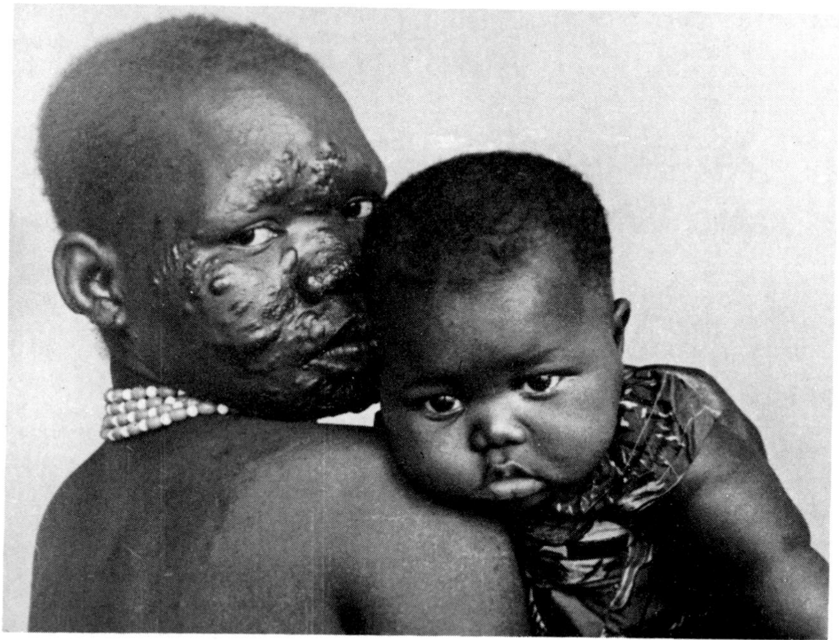

Fig. 1.1 It appears that the infant, like the great majority of infants born to mothers with lepromatous leprosy, has been protected by the placental barrier, but runs the risk of postnatal infection.

Infection via the skin

This has long been suspected, and with the rare exception of leprosy acquired by direct implantation of bacilli into the skin by tattoo or hypodermic needle, the two likely routes being direct skin-to-skin contact or transmission by flies and other arthropods. But microscopic examination of skin sections shows the presence of a clear and uninvolved zone immediately beneath the epidermis (the papillary zone), with bacilli favouring the deeper portions of the dermis (corium). Furthermore, very few bacilli, if any, are found in the epidermis or on the surface of intact skin.[2] Protagonists of the skin-to-skin hypothesis counter these arguments by citing the large numbers of bacilli that can be excreted by necrotising or ulcerating skin lesions, and although they cannot claim that bacilli are capable of penetrating intact skin, they can reasonably claim that they may enter via an abrasion. However, it is very unlikely that ulcerated skin would ever be rubbed against healthy skin, let alone abraded skin, and, in any case, bacilli found in necrotising skin lesions (erythema necroticans) are invariably dead. However, arthropods are capable of carrying leprosy bacilli, not only from the skin but also from nasal secretions. A detailed study[3] has shown that the legs, abdomen, mouth parts and faeces of flies are heavily contaminated with bacilli after feeding on nasal mucus and ulcerating skin lesions. Moreover, *M. leprae* can remain viable in desiccated nasal secretion for 1–7 days.[4] Biting insects are another potential danger as they are capable of collecting bacilli from the skin and transferring them when biting healthy skin. Transference of *M. leprae* from humans to mouse foot pads by mosquitoes has been demonstrated.[5] No final judgement can be made at this stage of our knowledge, but few would disagree with Rees[6] when he stresses the importance of controlling fly populations in and around leprosy units.

Infection via the gastrointestinal tract

Although it is known that leprosy bacilli can be conveyed to food by flies, and that they are present in the breast milk of mothers suffering from lepromatous leprosy, nothing is yet known about the risk of leprosy infection via the gastrointestinal tract.

Infection via the respiratory tract

Schäffer,[7] as long ago as 1898, made a careful study of the possible spread of leprosy by droplets (aerosols), and his paper has been translated from German into English. Recently, there has been a revival of interest in this subject, and investigations on the nasal mucosa[8] and on nasal mucus[9] in untreated lepromatous leprosy leave no doubt that infected droplets can be discharged into the atmosphere in the act of talking, sneezing or coughing, or can be absorbed by dust. Clearly, the risk of inhaling leprosy bacilli is greatly increased where living conditions are poor and overcrowding is the rule. Recent experimental work, in which immunologically suppressed mice were subjected to aerosols containing *M. leprae*,[10] has given strong support to this hypothesis, for 33% of the mice were infected by this means, and the presumption is that some of the many inspired leprosy bacilli could have entered capillaries in the alveoli of the lungs to be carried thence to sites suitable for multiplication. They are able to do this without causing lesions at the portals of entry, for no lesions were found in the respiratory tracts of these mice. Pallen and McDermott[11] have drawn attention to Barton's suggestion that the anterior end of the inferior turbinate is a possible site of entry of *M. leprae*,[8] and they add that nasal mucosal damage from the common cold may be a facilitating factor.

General considerations

The disease we know as leprosy, caused by *M. leprae*, can no longer be considered a disease confined to humans, for naturally-acquired leprosy has been reported in the armadillo, the chimpanzee and the Mangabey monkey; hence it has been labelled a zoonosis.[12] Furthermore, there has been a report of leprosy developing in five armadillo handlers in Texas, all native-born men and without any history of known contact with leprosy.[13] Humans, who are the most likely source of infection for other humans, or for susceptible animals, are those who harbour *M. leprae* in the upper respiratory tract, especially in the nose, and these probably constitute about 20% of all leprosy sufferers. But the proviso must be made that their disease is untreated, for effective chemotherapy renders leprosy bacilli non-viable relatively rapidly. *Danger to others, if any, arises not from the leprosy patient under treatment but from the undiagnosed case.*

Bad housing conditions and inadequate food are important factors in the spread of leprosy, for domestic overcrowding, particularly at night, provides the ideal conditions for infection whether by droplets or by skin contact, and under-nourishment reduces cell-mediated immunity (see Chapter 5). Campaigns to control leprosy in endemic regions should take these factors into account. It should be noted that Hansen, the discoverer of the leprosy bacillus, went to the USA in 1888 to see if he could find leprosy in the descendants of Norwegians who had emigrated from Norway in order to avoid segregation; he found no leprosy in these families and gave it as his opinion that this was largely due to good housing and living conditions.

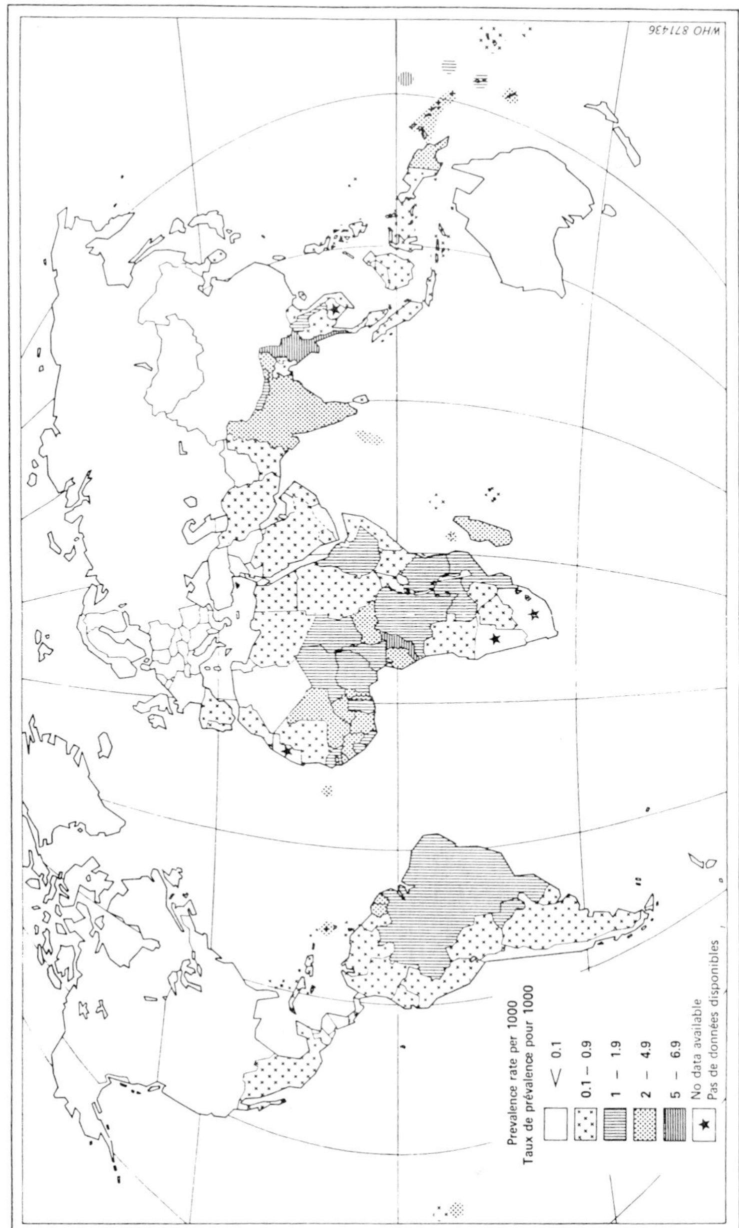

Fig. 1.2 Prevalence of registered leprosy cases in the world (1987). (This map was established by the leprosy unit of WHO and is reproduced with permission of the World Health Organization, Geneva.)

WORLD DISTRIBUTION, PAST AND PRESENT

Leprosy has a wide distribution in the world (Fig. 1.2), and is most prevalent in the tropics and subtropics, but it also occurs as an endemic disease, but less commonly, in temperate regions, such as the Mediterranean littoral, among the aborigines of Australia,[14] and in native-born US citizens resident in Texas and Louisiana.[15] The most recent authoritative estimate of the total number of cases in the world is 11.5 million, with at least 5 300 000 registered cases (Table 1.1).

Table 1.1 Epidemiology of leprosy in relation to control. (Report of a WHO Study Group (1982) Technical Report Series 675. Geneva: WHO)

WHO Region	*Year*	*Number of cases (thousands)*
Africa	(1975)	3500
America	(1975)	400
South-East Asia	(1981)	5350
Europe	(1975)	25
Eastern Mediterranean	(1981)	250
Western Pacific	(1975)	2000
Total		11 525

Leprosy is generally believed to have originated in Asia, and the earliest records of a leprosy-like disease come from China and India of the 6th century BC. In China, a disciple of Confucius named Pai-Niu suffered from a disease resembling lepromatous leprosy, which was known at that time as *lai, li* and *Ta Feng*.[16,17,18] Ma Haide gives *Da Feng* as the early name in China.[19] Lowe[20] records that in India leprosy was first described in the *Susruth Samhita*, written about 600 BC, and treatment with chaulmoogra oil was known at that time. Rastogi and Rastogi[21] quote the Sanscrit word *kustha* as the original name in India for leprosy. Hopes that the skulls and bones of Egyptian mummies might reveal even earlier evidence of leprosy have not been fulfilled; the earliest paleopathological evidence to date is in mummies of the 2nd century BC.[22] The disease was probably carried from India to Europe in the 4th century BC by returning soldiers and camp followers from the Greek wars of conquest in Asia, led by Alexander the Great, and the earliest description of a disease which was unmistakably leprosy was by Aretaeus, in Greece, about 150 AD. He called the disease elephantiasis. From Greece, leprosy slowly spread throughout Europe, conveyed by infected soldiers, traders and settlers, and in Western and Northern Europe the disease was most active between the 10th and 15th centuries. Richards, in his well illustrated book,[23] has made an outstanding contribution to our understanding of the leprosy situation in medieval Britain and Scandinavia, and Irgens[24] has described the history of leprosy in Norway dating from the middle of the 19th century, and reports that a little under 2 per 1000 Norwegians were known to have leprosy at that time (a prevalence of 16.7 per 10 000 over the whole country). Over the next half-century the disease underwent a steady and significant decline to 1 per 100 000 by the year 1900.[25] Any doubts that the disease in the Middle Ages was actually leprosy, as some medical historians have claimed, were dispelled by Møller-Christensen when he discovered in Naestved, Denmark, the burial ground of a lazar hospital which existed between 1250 and 1550 AD. He was able to demonstrate classical changes of leprosy in many of the skulls and bones which were excavated.[26] A visit to his museum (Leprosy Museum, 62 Bredgade, Copenhagen), forming part of the medical historical museum and containing his best osseous material, is an experience not to be missed.

The last indigenous case of leprosy in Britain was recorded in 1798 when John Berns, a Shetland islander, was admitted to Edinburgh Royal Infirmary. In Western and Northern Europe, leprosy is now an imported disease, but in Southern Europe the disease has persisted to the present day as a minor health problem and is proving difficult to eradicate. Descriptions of leprosy in Siberia[27] and in Scandinavia in the previous century disprove the commonly-held view that the disease needs a warm climate in which to flourish.

REFERENCES

1 Duncan M. E., Melsom R., Pearson M. H., Menzel S., Barnetson R. St C. (1983). A clinical and immunological study of four babies of mothers with lepromatous leprosy, two of whom developed leprosy in infancy. *International Journal of Leprosy*; **51**: 7–17.

2 Pedley J. C. (1970). Composite skin contact smears: a method

of demonstrating the non-emergence of *Mycobacterium leprae* from intact lepromatous skin. *Leprosy Review*; **41**: 31–43.

3 Geater J. G. (1975). The fly as potential vector in the transmission of leprosy. *Leprosy Review*; **46**: 279–86.

4 Davey T. F., Rees R. J. W. (1974). The nasal discharge in leprosy: clinical and bacteriological aspects. *Leprosy Review*; **45**: 121–34.

5 Narayanan E., Sreevatsa, Kirchheimer W. F., Bedi B. M. S. (1977). Transfer of leprosy bacilli from patients to mouse footpads by *Aedes aegypti. Leprosy in India*; **49**: 181–6.

6 Rees R. J. W. (1975). Do flies transmit leprosy? *Leprosy Review*; **46**: 255–6.

7 Schäffer I. (1898). On the spread of leprosy bacilli from the upper parts of the respiratory tract (in German, but the editor of *Leprosy Review* holds a translation). *Archives of Dermatology and Syphilology*; **44**: 159–74.

8 Barton R. P. E. (1974). A clinical study of the nose in lepromatous leprosy. *Leprosy Review*; **45**: 135–44.

9 Pedley J. C. (1973). The nasal mucus in leprosy. *Leprosy Review*; **44**: 33–5.

10 Rees R. J. W., McDougall A. C. (1976). Airborne infection with *Mycobacterium leprae* in mice. *International Journal of Leprosy*; **44**: 99–103.

11 Pallen M. J., McDermott R. D. (1986). How might *Mycobacterium leprae* enter the body? *Leprosy Review*; **57**: 289–97.

12 Walsh G. P., Meyers W. M., Binford C. H., Gerone P. J., Wolf R. H., Leininger J. R. (1981). Leprosy—a zoonosis. *Leprosy Review*; **52 (suppl. 1)**: 77–83.

13 Lumpkin L. R., Fox G. F., Wolf J. E. (1983). Leprosy in five armadillo handlers. *Journal of the American Academy of Dermatology*; **9**: 899–903.

14 Hargrave J. C. (1970). Leprosy in Northern Territory Aborigines. Canberra: Northern Territory Medical Service of the Australian Department of Health.

15 Binford C. H., Meyers W. M., Walsh G. P. (1982). Leprosy. *Journal of the American Medical Association*; **247**: 2283–92.

16 Skinsnes O. K. (1964). Leprosy in society. II. The pattern of concept and reaction to leprosy in oriental antiquity. *Leprosy Review*; **35**: 106–22.

17 Skinsnes O. K. (1980). Leprosy in archaeologically recovered

bamboo book in China. *International Journal of Leprosy*; **48**: 333.

18 Skinsnes O. K., Chang P. H. C. (1985). Understanding leprosy in ancient China. *International Journal of Leprosy*; **53**: 289–307.

19 Haide Ma, Ganyun Ye (1982). Leprosy work in China. *Leprosy Review*; **53**: 81–4.

20 Lowe J. (1947). Comments on the history of leprosy. *Leprosy Review*; **18**: 54–63.

21 Rastogi N., Rastogi R. C. (1984). Leprosy in ancient India. *International Journal of Leprosy*; **52**: 541–3.

22 Dzierzykray-Rogalski T. (1980). Paleopathology of the Ptolemaic inhabitants of Dakhleh Oasis (Egypt). *Journal of Human Evolution*; **9**: 71–4.

23 Richards P. (1977). *The Medieval Leper and his Northern Heirs*. Cambridge: D. S. Brewer.

24 Irgens L. M. (1980). Leprosy in Norway. *Leprosy Review*; **51 (suppl. 1)**.

25 Irgens L. M. (1981). Epidemiological aspects and implications of the disappearance of leprosy from Norway; some factors contributing to the decline. *Leprosy Review*; **52 (suppl. 1)**: 147–65.

26 Møller-Christensen V. (1978). *Leprosy Changes of the Skull*. Odense: Odense University Press.

27 Marsden K. (1892). *On Sledge and Horseback to Outcast Siberian Lepers*. London: The Record Press.

2 The Disease

BACTERIAL AND PATHOLOGICAL ASPECTS

The cause of leprosy is an acid-fast mycobacterium *Mycobacterium leprae (M. leprae)*, which is an obligate intracellular mycobacterium; the word 'obligate' implying that it is obligatory for it to live intracellularly. It has been found in many different types of cells, most commonly within macrophages but also within Schwann cells of nerves, muscle cells, lining endothelial cells of blood vessels, melanocytes of skin and chondrocytes of cartilage, to mention the most important. It is a single strain species (see p. 68) which, after staining, resembles *M. tuberculosis* in appearance under the microscope.

In stained skin slit-smears and sections it can be seen lying singly, in clumps, or in compact masses within macrophages; these are known as globi (Plate 1). The term 'acid-fast' refers to the capacity of the bacillus, when stained with a red dye (carbol fuchsin), to retain its red colour when treated with acid. Tubercle and leprosy bacilli are alcohol-fast as well as acid-fast, and a mixture of acid and alcohol is used in the standard method of staining – the Ziehl–Neelsen method. However, *M. leprae* is less acid- and alcohol-fast than *M. tuberculosis* is, and this fact is of practical importance when it comes to applying the Ziehl–Neelsen method of staining, for if it is used in leprosy in the same manner as in tuberculosis, it is likely that bacilli will not be found for the simple reason that the leprosy bacilli will have been decolourised and therefore will not be identifiable under the microscope. This problem is overcome by having a weaker acid–alcohol mixture and by leaving it in contact with the slide for a shorter time. In a properly stained skin smear the leprosy bacilli appear bright red and everything else takes the colour of the counter-stain used. If stained smears are treated with pyridine the bacilli lose their red colour; this is known as pyridine extractability,[1] and distinguishes *M. leprae* from all other pathogenic mycobacteria. (*M. vaccae* and *M. phlei* have been shown to lose their acid-fastness when extracted with pyridine,[2] but these are non-pathogenic mycobacteria.) Details of the structure of *M. leprae* have been given by Draper.[3]

Ziehl–Neelsen method of staining *M. leprae* in smears

There are many minor modifications of this method, each as good as another in the hands of an experienced technician, and the method described here is a reliable guide:

1 The slide with the smear on it should be covered with carbol fuchsin and heat applied beneath it, either with a gas flame (Bunsen burner) or with a spirit lamp. Heating should be sufficient to cause steam to rise from all parts of the slide, but boiling is avoided. The slide should be left for 15 minutes without any further heating.
2 The stain is tipped away and the slide is held under a gentle stream of water.
3 Pour acid–alcohol mixture on to the slide and leave for 3 seconds if the smear is thin or for 5 seconds if the smear is thick, then wash it away with running water. The acid–alcohol mixture consists of 1% hydrochloric acid in 70% alcohol. The slide is inspected to see the degree of pinkness; if faintly pink proceed to the next stage, but if deeply pink treat again with acid–alcohol for 2 seconds and wash with running water.
4 Cover the slide with counter-stain, such as 1% methylene blue for about 10 seconds.
5 Wash in running water and allow to dry.

Bacterial indices

It should be noted that *M. leprae*, in common with other mycobacteria, retains the property of staining with carbol fuchsin when no longer alive. Therefore, a technician examining skin smears during treatment will get the impression that the patient is making no progress unless he can differentiate living from dead bacilli. The morphology or structure of the bacilli seen after Ziehl–Neelsen staining is all-important, since living bacilli appear as uniformly stained rods (solid-staining) and dead bacilli appear irregularly stained (fragmented bacilli) or as granules (granular bacilli) (Plate 2). The density of bacilli in smears is known as the bacterial (bacteriological) index (BI) and includes both living and dead bacilli. It can be recorded in a number of ways, the simplest being a system recording many bacilli (+++), moderate numbers (++), few (+) and no bacilli (−). But if a more comprehensive system is desired, Ridley's logarithmic scale[4] is recommended. This is based on the number of bacilli seen in an average microscopic field using an oil-immersion objective ($^1/_{12}$ in or 2 mm) (Fig. 2.1):

6+ Many clumps of bacilli in an average field (over 1000).
5+ 100–1000 bacilli in an average field.
4+ 10–100 bacilli in an average field.
3+ 1–10 bacilli in an average field.
2+ 1–10 bacilli in 10 fields.
1+ 1–10 bacilli in 100 fields.

If several smears are taken, the mean index is calculated. In lepromatous patients under treatment it will be found that there will be no fall in the BI during the first 12 months because dead and living bacilli are being counted, since both are stained red by carbol fuchsin, but after this a steady fall takes place over the next 5–10 years. Clearly, a more sensitive index of bacteriological improvement is required for such patients; hence the introduction of a system of classifying the bacilli in smears into two groups, solid-stained (living) and irregularly-stained (dead).[5] Colour plate 2 shows the subdivision of non-viable bacilli into fragmented and granular. It should be noted that there is nothing new in considering granular bacilli to be dead; this view was originally put forward by Hansen in 1895.[6] The morphological index (MI) is the percentage of solid-stained bacilli, calculated after examining 200 red-staining elements *lying singly*, and a knowledge of this index will tell if a patient's leprosy is active or not, will give valuable information as to response to treatment, and will give early intimation of bacterial resistance to chemotherapy or of defaulting on treatment. That is to say, an increase in MI indicates a worsening of the patient's condition, and a decrease indicates improvement. In general, it can be said that the MI of lepromatous patients

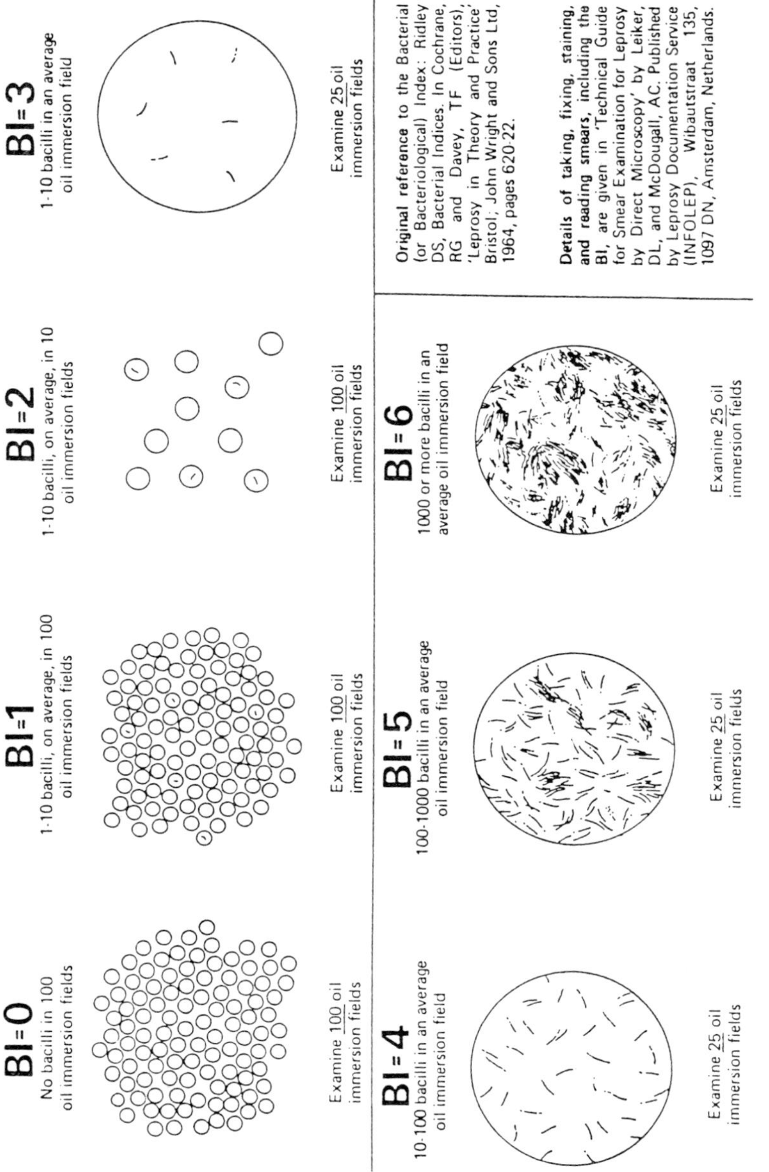

Fig. 2.1 Leprosy smears: bacterial (bacteriological) index (BI) — Ziehl–Neelsen stain.

commencing treatment will be somewhere between 25 and 75, and, whereas there is a steady fall in MI to zero in 4–6 months of dapsone monotherapy (Fig. 2.2), the fall is considerably more rapid with multidrug therapy.

Ridley prefers his SFG index[7] in which bacilli are divided into three classes: 'solid' (S), 'fragmented' (F) and 'granular' (G). A value is assigned to the bacilli of each class in a smear: 2 if they appear numerous (over 20% of all bacilli); 1 if few (1–20%); 0 if less than 1%. Thus, the relative proportion of bacilli in the three classes SFG (in this order) are represented by one of the permutations of 2–1–0. These combinations are placed in order of descending granularity from 2–0–0 (all solid) to 0–0–2 (all granular) to give an index as shown below:

SFG value		*SFG index*
2–0–0		10
2–1–0		9
2–2–0		8
2–1–1	(1–2–0)	7
2–2–1		6
1–2–1	(2–2–2)	5
1–2–2		4
1–1–2	(0–2–1)	3
0–2–2		2
0–1–2		1
0–0–2		0

If several smears are available the mean index is taken. An SFG index of 2 or less signifies that there are no solid-staining unbroken rods. The technique of making smears is described in Chapter 4, p. 60. Although the BI of a smear reflects the density of bacilli in a skin lesion, it gives no indication of the size of the lesion, hence Ridley devised a biopsy index which could not only show the bacterial density but also the size of the lesion.[8] Later he described the use of serial biopsies in therapeutic trials,[9] and a logarithmic index of bacilli in biopsies.[10]

Mycobacterium leprae was discovered by Hansen in Norway in 1873 and his observations were published in 1874;[11] therefore, if we except *Pseudomonas aeruginosa* and *Bacillus anthracis*, it is the oldest known bacterium pathogenic to man. Yet it has consistently defied cultivation on artificial media, attempts to infect volunteers

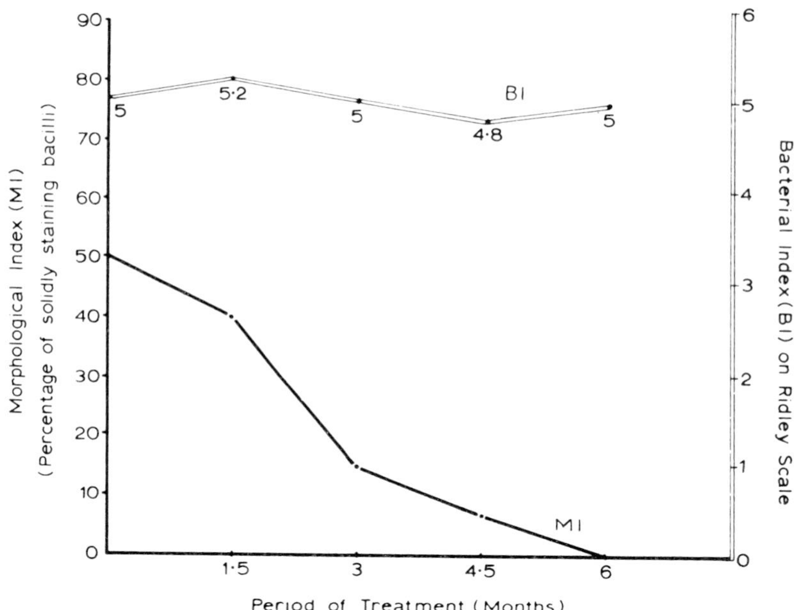

Fig. 2.2 Effect of treatment on BI and MI.

have all failed, and only since 1960 have techniques been developed for the transmission of leprosy to animals. Shepard [12] was the first to succeed in growing *M. leprae* in a laboratory animal. He chose the foot pads of mice because of their cool temperature (as many had done before him) but he succeeded because he counted the numbers of bacilli injected; he found that inocula had to contain less than 10^6 bacilli (1 million), and obtained the best multiplication with inocula of about 10^3 (1000) bacilli. These infections remained localised to the foot pad, and it was not until 1966 that a disseminated infection was obtained by Rees[13] in immature mice previously treated by thymectomy and whole-body irradiation to depress their immunity.

Whatever the route of entry into the human body, only a proportion of persons infected develop signs of the disease after the usual incubation period of 3–5 years. The majority develop a sub-clinical infection, and this has been shown by immunologists investigating leprosy contacts for evidence of cell-mediated immunity to *M. leprae*.[14] Biopsies from persons who have been in contact with leprosy patients have sometimes shown the presence of a single bacillus in skin, muscle or nerve, yet no signs of leprosy have developed during subsequent follow-up examinations. In the case of a susceptible host, the type of leprosy which will develop is determined by the way in which the defensive cells respond to the challenge once they have 'recognised' the infection. The first testing place is likely to be within peripheral nerves, for leprosy bacilli have a predilection for neural tissue and whatever may be the route of entry into nerves the target organ is the Schwann cell.[15] Once bacilli have been engulfed by Schwann cells their subsequent fate, and the type of leprosy which ensues, depend on the resistance of the infected individual (Chapter 5). Resistance is highest in tuberculoid leprosy (TT), diminishes through the borderline spectrum, and is lowest in lepromatous leprosy (LL) (see Fig. 2.4).

Not only do leprosy bacilli have a predilection for nerves but they are the only bacteria to have the capacity to enter nerves. Although it has yet to be proved, it is suspected that they do so via endoneurial blood vessels.[16] The endoneurium is the fine layer of tissue enclosing Schwann cells and axons, and a group of these minute structures are enclosed by a multilayered tissue known as perineurium to form a nerve fascicle (Fig. 2.3). Alternative names are fasciculus and funiculus. The epineurium is the outer coat of a nerve and is a loose connective tissue sheath binding the fascicles together.

Nerves invaded by leprosy bacilli are either dermal (cutaneous) nerves or nerve trunks, and the two regions which are most vulnerable are where the nerves are most cool and where they are subject to trauma; often these two factors coincide.

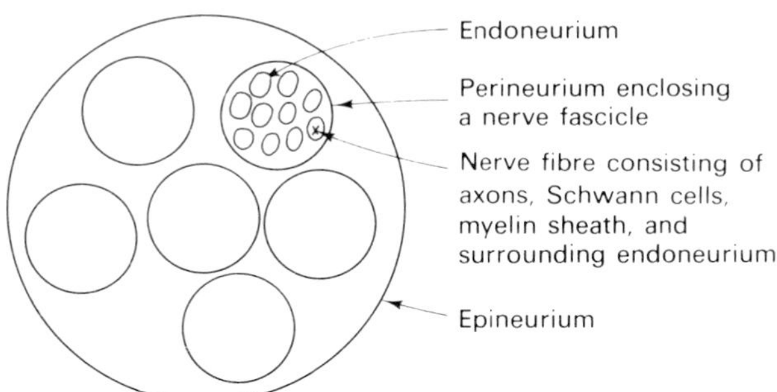

Fig. 2.3 Diagrammatic representation of a cross-section of a peripheral nerve.

TUBERCULOID LEPROSY (TT)

Bacilli which enter Schwann cells multiply within them and slowly destroy them; the process is slow because of the 12–13 days taken by each bacillus to divide into two. Bacilli liberated by effete Schwann cells enter neighbouring Schwann cells and thus the intraneural infection spreads, but a stage is reached when the intraneural infection is 'recognised' and the nerve is invaded by lymphocytes and histiocytes (macrophages); the latter become fixed epithelioid cells, and groups of these become giant cells. Thus, the tuberculoid granuloma is formed and leads to the nerve's destruction, and this in turn results in anaesthesia and/or muscle weakness, depending on the type of nerve involved. In the case of a nerve trunk, such as the ulnar nerve for example, the enlargement of the affected part of the nerve, caused by the granuloma within it, occurs where the nerve is nearest the surface of the body[17] where it is coolest and most liable to trauma, and nerve thickening can readily be palpated. Pain may be present in the earlier stages of the destructive process, possibly in the absence of signs of nerve dysfunction, for it must be remembered that about 30% of the sensory fibres must be destroyed before evidence of sensory impairment can be detected. If the body's defence mechanism (cell-mediated immunity) is capable of anchoring the infection within one or more nerves, without evidence of skin involvement, this is referred to as pure neural tuberculoid leprosy.[18] But if bacilli or their antigens escape from the nerve into surrounding or neighbouring skin, a skin lesion is likely to develop at that site, and a biopsy of the lesion will reveal a tuberculoid granuloma which tends to collect in foci surrounding neurovascular elements, each focus consisting of epithelioid cells at the centre with a surrounding zone of lymphocytes (round cells); giant cells are sometimes present among the epithelioid cells (Plate 3). Some of these foci invade the papillary zone of the skin immediately beneath the epidermis – the zone which is always free in lepromatous and borderline leprosy – and may even erode the basal layer of the epidermis. Bacilli will not be seen. Dermal nerves within the tuberculoid foci are either completely destroyed (and therefore are unrecognisable), or appear greatly swollen by epithelioid cell granuloma and surrounded by a zone of lymphocytes: occasionally, there may be caseation within a dermal nerve.[19]

BORDERLINE LEPROSY (BT, BB and BL)

The name 'borderline' has replaced the earlier name 'dimorphous'. Nerves are attacked in the same way as described for TT but higher concentrations of bacilli are required to elicit a cellular response, depending on the position of the patient in the borderline spectrum (see Fig. 2.4). The cellular response is less focal and less destructive, and microscopic examination reveals zones of epithelioid cells adjacent to areas of bacillated Schwann cells. Some epithelioid cell foci will be found next to, or within, the perineurium. Bacilli will be found within affected nerves, in small numbers at the tuberculoid end of the spectrum and in large numbers at the lepromatous end. Clinical evidence of nerve damage, whether sensory or motor, or both, is likely to antedate skin lesions by months or years, and in one case polyneuritic symptoms and signs persisted for 8 years before skin lesions were noted.[20] Histological examination of a skin lesion in borderline leprosy shows characteristic features. In *borderline-tuberculoid leprosy* (BT) there is an epithelioid cell granuloma more diffuse than in TT with a free, but narrow, papillary zone. Giant cells tend to be of foreign body type rather than of Langhans type, and dermal nerves are moderately swollen by cellular infiltrate or may show only Schwann cell proliferation. Bacilli are usually absent from the dermis, but a few are likely to be found within dermal nerves. In *mid-borderline leprosy* (BB) there is a diffuse epithelioid cell granuloma with scanty lymphocytes and no giant cells. The papillary zone is clear and dermal nerves show slight swelling and cellular infiltrate. Bacilli are present within the dermis and within dermal nerves in moderate numbers. In *borderline-lepromatous leprosy* (BL) there is a macrophage granuloma in which some of the cells may show slight foamy change, and lymphocytes are present in dense clumps or are widely distributed in parts of the granuloma; a few epithelioid cells occasionally may be seen. Dermal nerves contain some cellular infiltrate and sometimes the perineurium has a peculiar laminated appearance known as 'onion-skin' perineurium. The papillary zone is clear, leprosy bacilli are plentiful, distributed singly or in clumps, and sometimes in small globi (bacilli massed within distended macrophages).

LEPROMATOUS LEPROSY (LL)

Because of depressed cell-mediated immunity, bacilli which enter Schwann cells multiply unchecked; they also enter perineurial cells to multiply within them, and subsequent perineurial damage has been described by Pearson and Ross.[16] Bacillary multiplication within perineurial cells impairs the competence of the perineurium to stabilise the intraneural environment, and the 'onion-peel' appearance which develops in a dermal nerve is due to infiltration of the perineurium with histiocytes and plasma cells. This type of nerve damage in lepromatous leprosy, secondary to perineurial damage, is different from the pathological process in the other types of leprosy and is much slower to unfold. In addition to the bacilli which multiply within Schwann cells and perineurial cells there are those which are liberated when these cells are destroyed; they are engulfed by histiocytes which, instead of destroying them and becoming fixed epithelioid cells (as they do in TT), become wandering macrophages. These allow bacilli to multiply within them while travelling to other parts of the nerve and to other nerves and tissues via blood, lymph and tissue fluid. These swollen macrophages, packed with bacilli, are known as lepra (*syn.* Virchow) cells, and the masses of bacilli which accumulate in their cytoplasm are called globi when seen in skin smears or biopsies.

Physical signs in the skin and nasal mucosa are likely to be noticed by the patient before signs of nerve damage are noticed, hence pure neural lepromatous leprosy has never been described. Once bacilli are liberated into the skin by the rupture of overstretched lepra cells, they are picked up by fresh histiocytes which similarly act as culture media while carrying their bacterial load to other skin areas or to distant tissues. If a skin section stained by haematoxylin and eosin (H & E) is examined under the microscope one sees thinning of the epidermis and flattening of rete ridges, there is a clear zone immediately beneath the epidermis (the papillary layer), whilst deeper in the dermis lies the typical diffuse leproma consisting of histiocytes and/or macrophages with, in addition, a few lymphocytes and plasma cells. Fragmented and granular bacilli within macrophages are responsible for their foamy appearance, and this is due to the presence of fat within macrophages. In sections stained to show bacilli (e.g. Fite–Faraco method of staining), bacilli packed within macrophages appear in dense rounded collections known as globi, while other bacilli are scattered singly or in small groups (Plate 1). Due to the extraordinary paradox that leprosy bacilli do not secrete toxins, the patient harbouring countless millions of bacilli can feel perfectly fit. Hanks[21] has calculated that the number of bacilli within 1 cm^3 of infiltrated skin, in a lepromatous subject, varies between 1 and 7 billion; the mean of 6 patients was 2.5 billion. Knowing the long generation time of *M. leprae* it seems incredible that there can be such a build-up of bacilli in the space of a few years. But, with a pencil and paper one can calculate that, even with a generation time of about 12 days, one bacillus will become 100 million by the end of 1 year! This is, of course, a purely theoretical figure, for even under the ideal conditions for multiplication existing in the lepromatous patient, some bacilli must die before being able to divide into two. Tissues bearing the brunt of the disease are: nerves; skin; eyes; reticuloendothelial system (this system includes lymph nodes and specialised cells of liver, spleen, and bone marrow); mucosa of mouth, nose, pharynx, larynx, and trachea; endothelium of small blood vessels; involuntary (plain) muscle, such as arrector pili and dartos; skeletal (voluntary) muscle; and, in the male, testes. As regards the nervous system, bacilli may reach the posterior root ganglia and the sympathetic ganglia, but are not found in spinal cord or brain. The disease is usually well established by the time lepromatous leprosy is diagnosed, and details of histological changes in nerves at this stage of the disease have been described by Job and Desikan.[22] It should be noted that fibrosis of nerves is an inevitable end-result of lepromatous leprosy in spite of chemotherapy if treatment has been commenced late in the course of the disease. This may lead to a peripheral and distinctive form of anaesthesia in arms and legs which is generally referred to as 'glove and stocking' anaesthesia. But this term is strictly inaccurate as the anaesthesia is not usually evenly distributed; it tends to be somewhat patchy due to the fact that the degree of damage to dermal nerves is not evenly distributed, and one reason for this may be *M. leprae*'s preference for the cooler sites. Those fortunate patients who are diagnosed at an early stage, when there is a manageable intraneural bacillary load, remain entirely free from sensory or motor deficit. As the disease responds to treatment, the leproma in the dermis shows increased foamy change, with vacuolation, and breaks up into discrete foci with

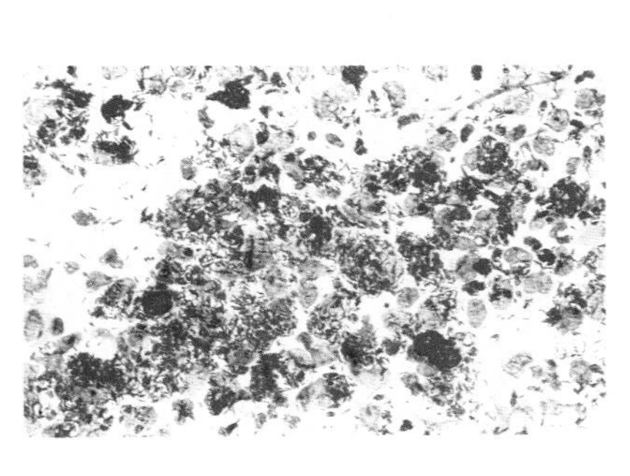

1

Plate 1 Leprosy bacilli seen in skin smear in lepromatous leprosy. B1=6.

Plate 2 Diagrammatic representation of various forms of *M. leprae* stained by modified Ziehl – Neelsen method.

Plate 3 Skin biopsy in tuberculoid leprosy stained by H & E. Note the lymphocytes (L), epithelioid cell (E) and Langhans giant cells (E) and Langhans giant cells (G). (Dr D. S. Ridley, Hospital for Tropical Diseases.)

Plate 4 Biopsy of a BT skin lesion showing leprosy bacilli within a dermal nerve (→). Smears from the lesion were negative. (Dr D. S. Ridley, Hospital for Tropical Diseases).

Plate 5 Tuberculoid leprosy. The only skin lesion present. Note its scaliness and dryness. It was insensitive, and the Mitsuda reaction was three-plus (+++).

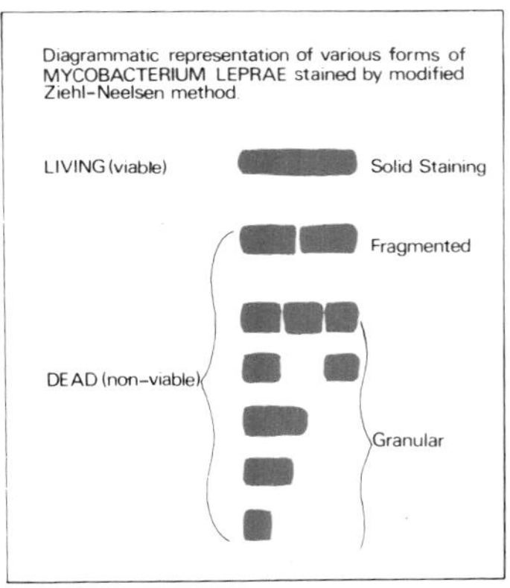

2

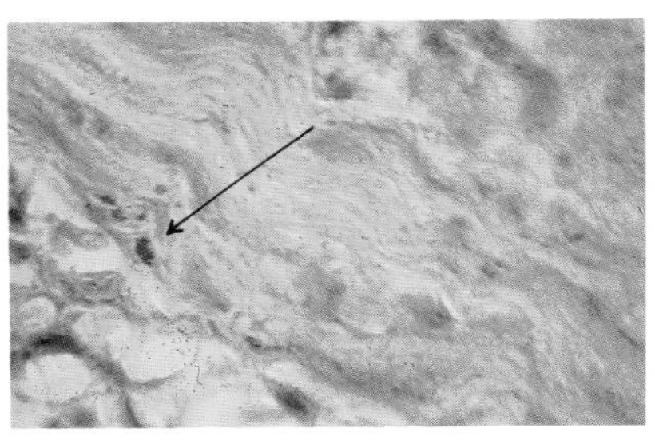

4

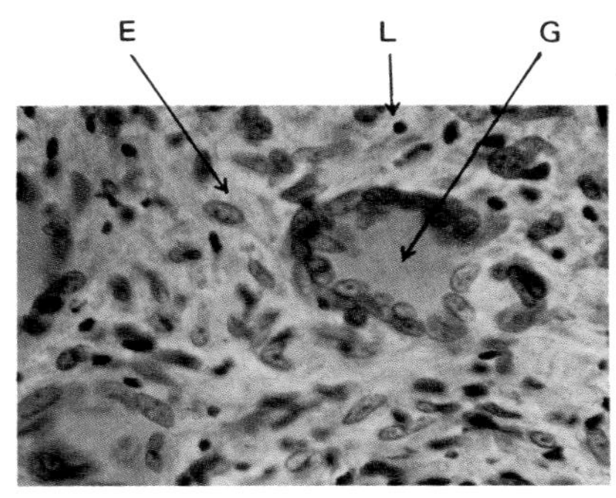

3

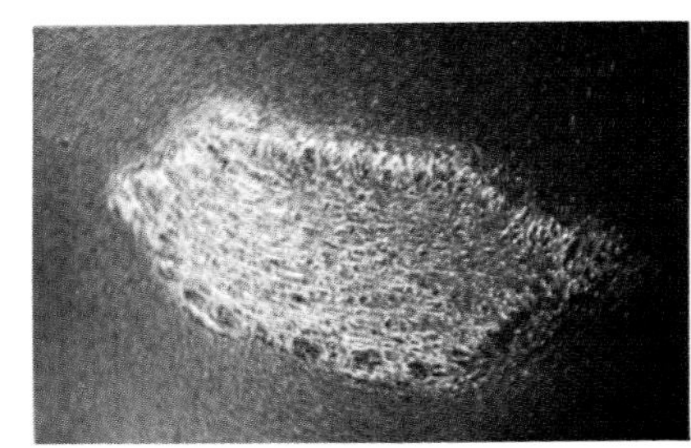

5

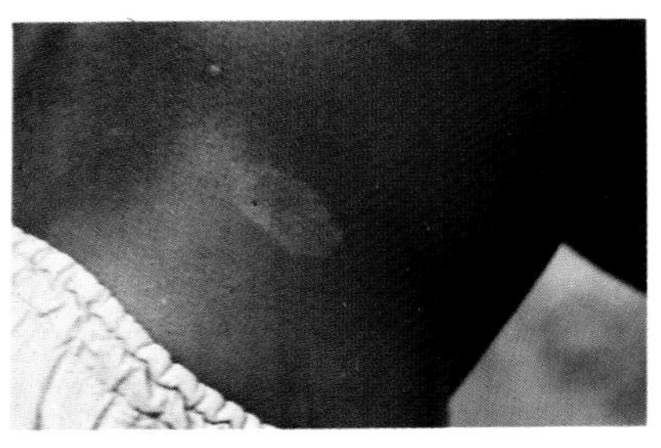

6

Plate 6 Hypopigmented macule of indeterminate leprosy. (Dr D. Harman.)

Plate 7 Annular lesions in borderline tuberculoid (BT) leprosy. The lesions showed moderate sensory loss, AFB were absent, and the Mitsuda reaction was one-plus (+).

Plate 8 Thickened supraorbital branch of trigeminal nerve (5th cranial nerve).

Plate 9 Punched-out lesions in mid-borderline (BB) leprosy. Lesions showed slight anaesthesia, AFB were present in moderate numbers, and the Mitsuda reaction was negative.

Plate 10 Active borderline lepromatous (BL) leprosy. The large, shiny, faintly hypopigmented macules showed slight sensory impairment, and smears from the macules were strongly positive.

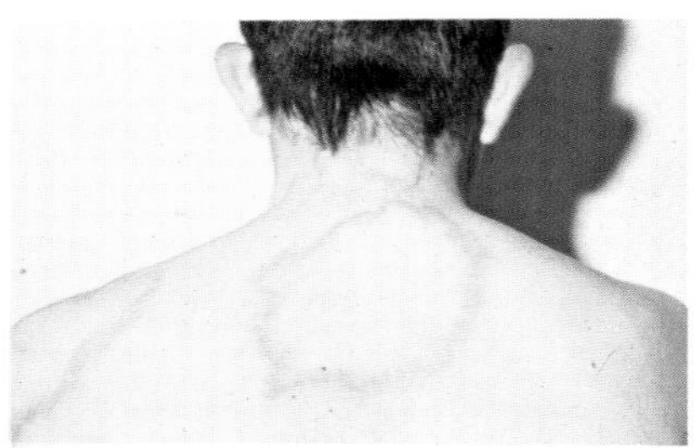

7

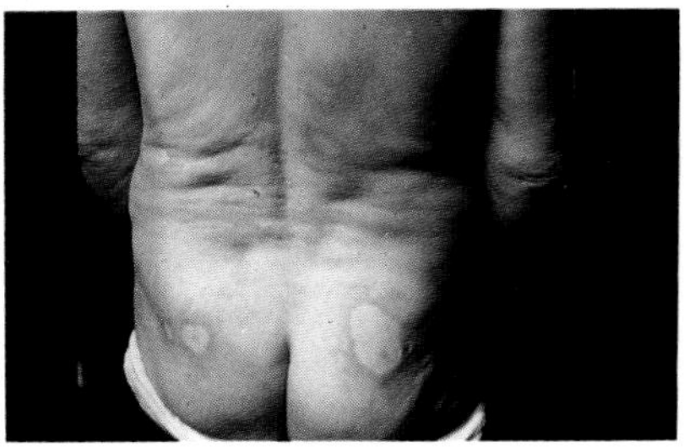

9

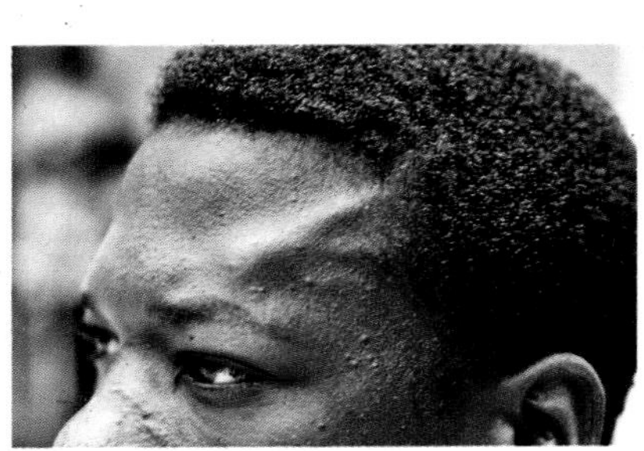

8

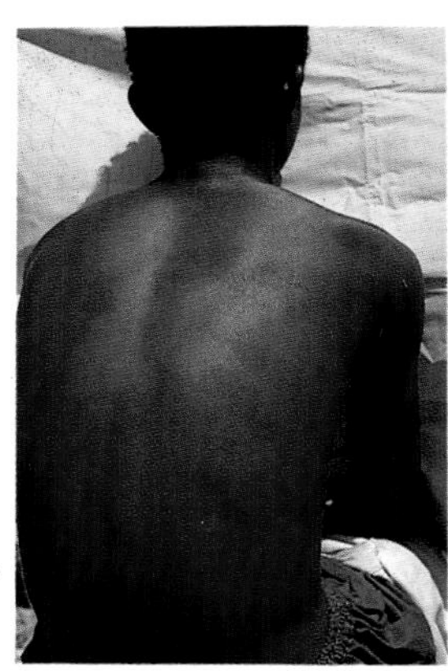

10

fibroblasts at the periphery. These foci shrink as treatment is continued; at the same time, bacilli in these foci become fragmented and granular.

A second edition of D. S. Ridley's *Skin Biopsy in Leprosy* was published in 1985, and individual copies are available on application to Pharma International, Ciba–Geigy Ltd., CH–4002 Basel, Switzerland.

INDETERMINATE LEPROSY (I)

This early and transitory stage of leprosy is found in persons (usually children) whose immunological status has yet to be determined. Histologically, there is a scattered non-specific histiocytic and lymphocytic infiltration which is diagnosable as leprosy in those cases in which there is a cellular reaction within a dermal nerve, or one or more leprosy bacilli are found in a situation, such as a dermal nerve, the subepidermal zone, or arrectores pilorum muscles. The latter are small involuntary muscles supplying hair follicles with erectile power.

HAEMATOLOGY AND SEROLOGY

A mild anaemia, which is normocytic and normochromic, and a raised erythrocyte sedimentation rate (ESR) are classical findings in LL. Impaired platelet adhesiveness and platelet aggregation to collagen, more pronounced in LL than in TT, has been demonstrated[23] and it has been suggested that the increased prothrombin time, commonly found in LL, is due to a circulating anticoagulant which is an IgM immunoglobulin.[24] Immunological abnormalities, such as raised levels of certain immunoglobulins, are discussed in Chapter 5, but in LL there are two serological abnormalities which are best described here. First, certain tests for syphilis may give a biological false-positive reaction in up to 60% of cases, namely, the Wassermann reaction (WR) – which registers anticardiolipin antibodies – and flocculation tests, such as the rapid plasma reagin test and the automated reagin test. The introduction of specific tests for syphilis, such as the *Treponema pallidum* haemagglutination assay test, has eliminated this problem. Second, tests used in the diagnosis of autoimmune disease may be positive in some cases, but results vary with geography and race (for example, tests for rheumatoid factor, LE cells, thyroglobulin antibodies, antispermatozoa antibodies, antinuclear factor, and cold precipitable protein).

CLINICAL ASPECTS OF LEPROSY

The most remarkable thing about leprosy is the enormously wide variation in the way the disease affects different persons; in some the disease involves only one peripheral nerve (a mononeuritis), or causes a single skin blemish which persists indefinitely or disappears of its own accord, while in others it produces countless nodules and other types of skin lesions, together with polyneuritis and damage to vital organs, such as eyes, larynx, testes and bones. Every conceivable variation occurs between these two extremes. The explanation lies in the infected individual's immune status (resistance)[25] (Fig. 2.4), and the fact that it is not a question of bacterial strains of varying pathogenicity has been confirmed by Rees[26] who has shown that leprosy bacilli from patients with different types of leprosy all behave in the same way when injected into susceptible mice. Doctors who are not engaged in leprosy work may fail to diagnose it unless they think of the possibility of the disease when confronted by a patient suffering from a skin disorder, for leprosy lesions cannot be diagnosed from their appearance alone and can be mimicked by a number of skin diseases. It is worth remembering that a combination of skin *and* neural disorder is strongly indicative of leprosy, and the correct diagnosis can

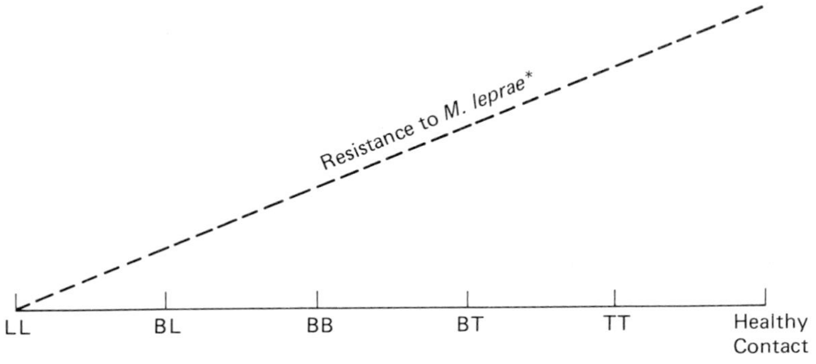

Fig. 2.4 The spectrum of immunity in leprosy.
Resistance = Interplay of cell-mediated immunity (CMI) and delayed hypersensitivity (DH).[27]

usually be made with the help of a pin and a scalpel; if a skin lesion is found to be insensitive, leprosy can confidently be suspected, and if the pin fails to demonstrate any sensory impairment, a smear can be made with the scalpel (see Chapter 4) and *M. leprae* may be found after suitable staining.

Lepromatous leprosy

It is unusual to have the opportunity to examine a patient in the early stages of lepromatous leprosy (unless there has been an earlier borderline phase which has attracted attention), as there are no symptoms of nerve involvement and early skin lesions are not likely to be noticed by the patient. This is doubly unfortunate, for not only is he infectious and therefore a potential danger to the public health, but he is missing the opportunity to have his disease arrested in the shortest possible time and to remain, so long as treatment is continued, free from the deformities of face and limbs which are the permanent hallmarks of late diagnosis. There are two symptoms which can alert the observant leprosy worker to a possible early diagnosis of lepromatous leprosy, and they may precede the classical skin lesions by months or years. Unfortunately, however, the patient is unlikely to make any mention of them unless specifically asked; these are nasal symptoms and oedema of legs. Nasal symptoms consist of stuffiness, crust formation, and blood-stained discharge. Nasal scraping, or nasal mucus (nose-blow), will reveal large numbers of bacilli; incidentally, a skin smear at this time, taken from apparently normal skin, will also be positive. Oedema of legs and ankles, always bilateral, is likely to be noted towards the end of the day, disappearing after a night's rest; only in the late stages is it persisent, and the legs become wooden hard on palpation. Oedema is due to a combination of gravity and increased capillary permeability, and the latter is probably due to a combination of leprous involvement of capillary endothelium and damage to autonomic fibres within dermal nerves controlling capillaries. McDougall and Archibald have described a patient who presented with oedema of legs and nasal symptoms, and was found to have active lepromatous leprosy.[28]

As for skin manifestations, patients may present with macules, papules, nodules, or with all three, but macules are likely to appear

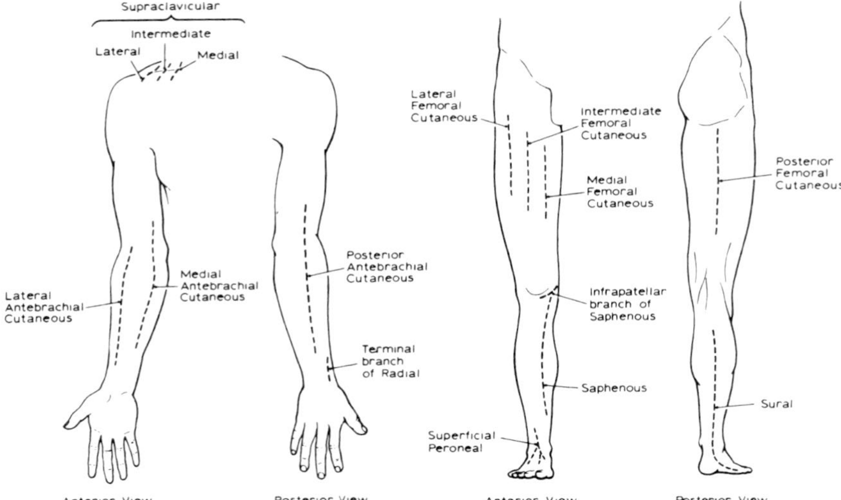

Fig. 2.5a and b **a** = Sensory nerves: arms; **b** = Sensory nerves: legs. (Note: mixed sensory and motor nerves are excluded.)

first. Skin lesions are multiple and have a distribution which is bilateral and symmetrical. Although face, arms, buttocks and legs are principally involved, the trunk may also be affected. Certain regions of the skin which have the highest temperatures are invariably spared, such as axillae, groins, perineum, and hairy scalp, thus conforming to the general rule that leprosy bacilli favour cooler temperatures. The scanty reports of leprosy lesions developing on the scalp all refer to the bald scalp, and the explanation of this discrepancy is that the skin temperature of the bald scalp is cooler temperatures. The scanty reports of leprosy lesions developing on the scalp all refer to the bald scalp, and the explanation of in the body. The diligent research worker will find small numbers of bacilli in smears or biopsies from the hairy scalp, in contrast to the enormous numbers present in the favoured skin areas, and even a few faint macules after shaving the patient's head, but he will not find plaques or nodules. *Macules* in lepromatous leprosy are erythematous on light skins, and on dark skins are coppery or may appear hypopigmented with a faint erythematous or coppery sheen. They are difficult to see but become more obvious when the patient becomes heated, e.g. after exercise on a hot day or after a hot bath. They are small, numerous, have a shiny surface and

become thinned by rarefying osteitis known as 'concentric bone atrophy', so that eventually only a fine needle of bone is left; this may disappear, in turn causing shortening of the affected toe or toes. In the metatarsals the first and most pronounced change takes place at the distal ends, usually commencing in the fifth metatarsal, the affected bones becoming thin and pointed – an appearance known as 'pencilling' or the 'sucked candy stick' (Fig. 2.10). Tarsal bone disintegration is an important yet often neglected cause of foot deformity and disability, and Grace Warren's paper[40] is essential reading. The factors responsible for these changes in hands and feet are multiple, and include various combinations of the following:

1 Repeated trauma because of absence of pain sensation. In the hands the terminal phalanges are most exposed to trauma, and in the feet the heads of the metatarsals bear the brunt because of the thrusting action of the rear foot driving the body forward when walking.
2 Impaired blood supply to bones due to endarteritis of nutrient vessels during lepra reaction.

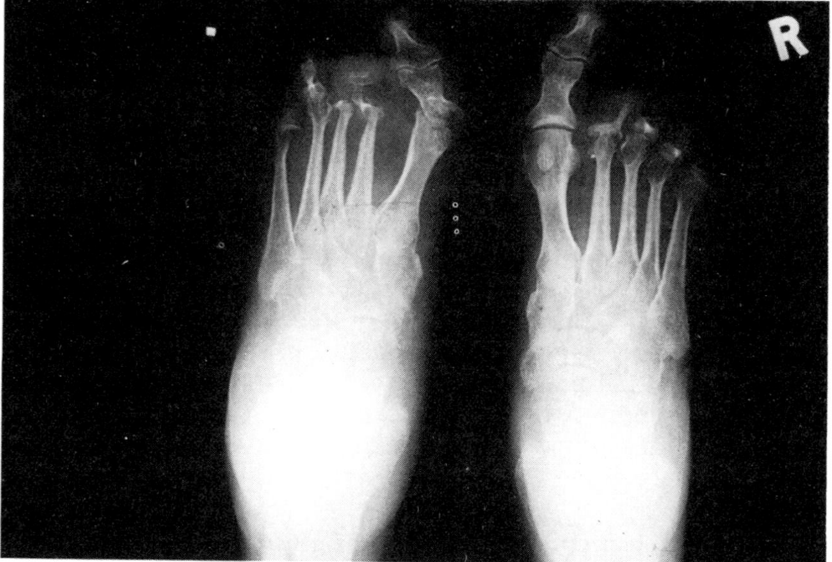

Fig. 2.10 X-ray of feet in lepromatous leprosy. Note 'pencilling' of some metatarsals, loss of several toes of both feet, and deformity of remaining toes. Both feet insensitive.

3 Impaired nerve supply to bones.
4 Deposition of leprosy bacilli in bones via the blood stream. (In advanced cases bacillary deposits cause leprous osteitis, giving finger phalanges a cystic appearance on x-ray.)
5 In males, generalised bone osteoporosis due to testicular atrophy and defective production of testosterone.
6 Disuse osteoporis may affect hand or foot due to paralysis and/or contractures causing reduced osteoblastic activity.
7 Osteomyelitis complicating chronic ulceration of the overlying skin.

It should be noted that whereas all the above-mentioned factors are operative in lepromatous leprosy, only 1, 3, 6 and 7 apply in non-lepromatous leprosy. The main reason why shortened fingers are characteristic of the former is that the hands of lepromatous patients may be insensitive for years before they become weak and therefore they are used in daily work, whereas in non-lepromatous patients anaesthesia and muscle weakness tend to occur together and paralysis of intrinsic muscles is rapid; therefore the affected hand is not used.

In the skull, two pathognomonic changes take place, namely, atrophy of the anterior nasal spine and of the maxillary alveolar process. The former contributes to nasal collapse and the latter causes loosening or loss of the upper central incisor teeth or of all four upper incisors, and these two skull changes have been given the name 'facies leprosa'.[31,32]

Testes

Varying degrees of testicular atrophy are likely to occur, particularly if the disease is neglected or if the treated patient undergoes repeated attacks of acute epididymo-orchitis during lepra reactions. In the earlier stages of testicular atrophy the patient remains sexually potent but his semen is devoid of spermatozoa and therefore he is sterile; impotence and gynaecomastia are later developments. Note that female reproductive organs are not affected in

Kidneys

Renal damage is an important cause of morbidity and mortality, yet it is not directly related to the disease (i.e. it is non-specific).

Non-specific pathology includes renal amyloidoisis, glomerulonephritis, interstitial nephritis, pyelonephritis and renal tuberculosis. Renal amyloidosis is subject to geographical variation, for it has been reported to occur in nearly 50% of patients in North America and in 80% in Spain. However, a low incidence is reported from Japan and India. Fortunately, the majority of these non-specific lesions are either self-limiting or will resolve with correct treatment, and this has been demonstrated in a random study of 35 lepromatous patients in India in various stages of treatment.[42] Renal biopsies revealed histological lesions in 16 patients (46%); 13 had proliferative glomerulonephritis in various stages of resolution, 2 had amyloidosis, and 1 had interstitial nephritis. Only in the last-mentioned case was renal damage considered to be irreversible. Desikan and Job[43] in their post-mortem study in India of different types of leprosy found that 11% of deaths were due to renal failure. But, it is likely that this figure is higher in Europe and North America because of the higher incidence of renal amyloidosis. The role of colchicine in controlling renal amyloidosis in chronic infections is under investigation.[44]

Muscles

There have been many reports of histological examination of skeletal muscles, tender and non-tender, but few of palpable nodules within muscles. A patient of one of the authors, 1 month after commencing treatment of LL, complained of difficulty in walking because of stiffness and discomfort in legs and thighs. On palpation there were firm, well-defined, non-tender masses of various sizes within affected muscles, and biopsy revealed extensive interstitial myositis with granular bacilli between muscle bundles.[45] Muscle biopsies in borderline cases have demonstrated granulomas containing macrophages and lymphocytes, but no bacilli.

Lymph nodes

Although lymph nodes have been reported to be moderately enlarged, in the authors' experience enlargement which can be detected clinically is confined to phases of lepra reaction and then there is marked swelling and tenderness, especially of femoral and inguinal groups.

Causes of death in leprosy

The causes of death in the vast majority of leprosy patients are the same as in the general population from which they are drawn, with the exception of renal damage in lepromatous leprosy. These renal complications are mostly self-limiting, but sometimes may result in chronic renal dysfunction leading to death from uraemia or from hypertension. A few additional comments must be made:

1 It is probable that in leprosy there is a reduced mortality from malaria because of the protection afforded by regular doses of dapsone.
2 There is a probable increased mortality from the side-effects of antileprosy drugs or from drugs used in the treatment of reactional states.
3 There is an increased mortality from severe lepra reaction, either from toxaemia if the reacting lesions are necrotic or from asphyxia resulting from glottic oedema. The post-mortem study of Desikan and Job found that 21.6% of deaths were from severe reactions.[43]
4 Mortality from cancer is no higher in leprosy patients than in the general population (see Chapter 5, p. 72).
5 The increased incidence of pulmonary tuberculosis observed in leprosaria gave rise to the presumption that leprosy patients were prone to tuberculosis. This view is no longer tenable, for it has been shown that it is no more common in leprosy outpatients than in the general population.[46]
6 There is an increased mortality from suicide.
7 In a number of papers mention has been made of the rarity of tetanus in leprosy patients in spite of the fact that anaesthesia of limbs is often complicated by chronic ulcers and injuries acquired at work. However, we would like to draw attention to the report of Desikan and Job,[43] who found that 13% of deaths in their series were due to tetanus, and to a recent report of tetanus complicating leprosy.[47]

Before moving on to a clinical description of other types of leprosy there are two manifestations of lepromatous leprosy requiring description.

Histoid leproma

This term, introduced by Wade,[48] is applied to the firm, erythematous, round or oval, shiny, glistening nodules, which appear on the

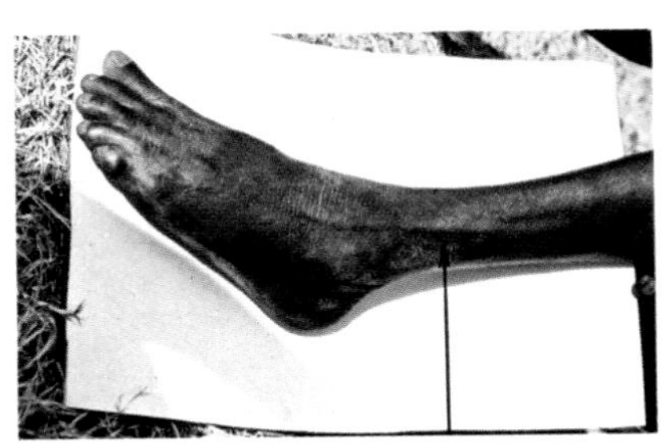

11

Plate 11 Thickened superficial peroneal nerve made more prominent by plantar-flexing the foot.

Plate 12 Early lepromatous leprosy. Note the small papular lesions distributed bilaterally and symmetrically. Similar lesions were present on face, buttocks and leg.

Plate 13 Superficial punctate keratitis in lepromatous leprosy. (Mr D. P. Choyce, Hospital for Tropical Diseases.)

Plate 14 Subpolar lepromatous leprosy (LLs). Note active papulonodules (recent) and plaques of boarderline leprosy (old-standing).

Plate 15 Secondary ichthyosis of the thigh in a patient who had been treated for lepromatous leprosy for many years. Both thighs, arms and lower legs were involved.

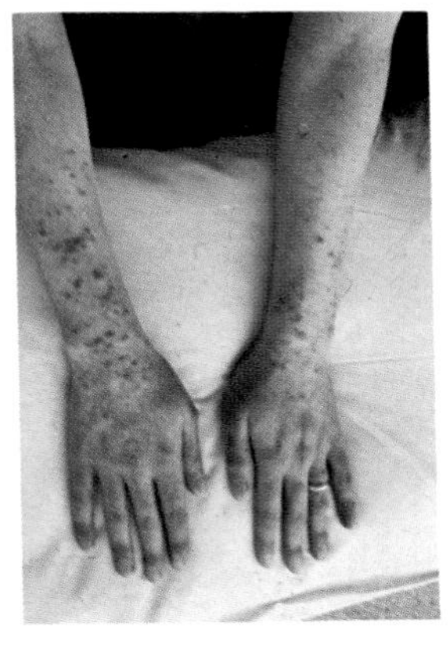

12

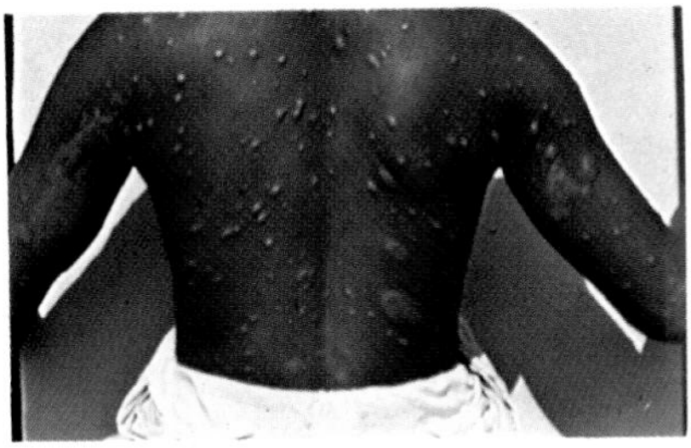

14

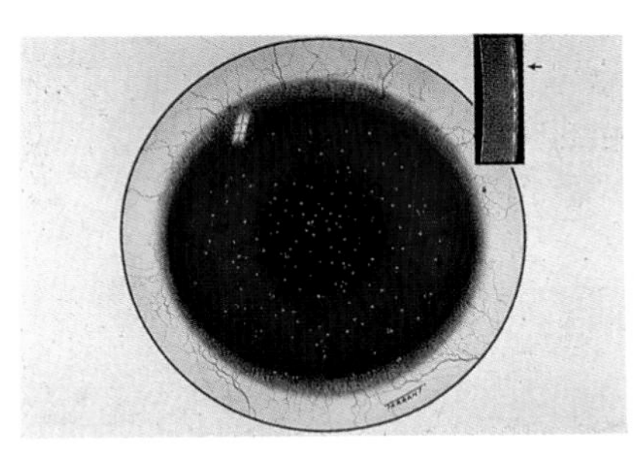

13

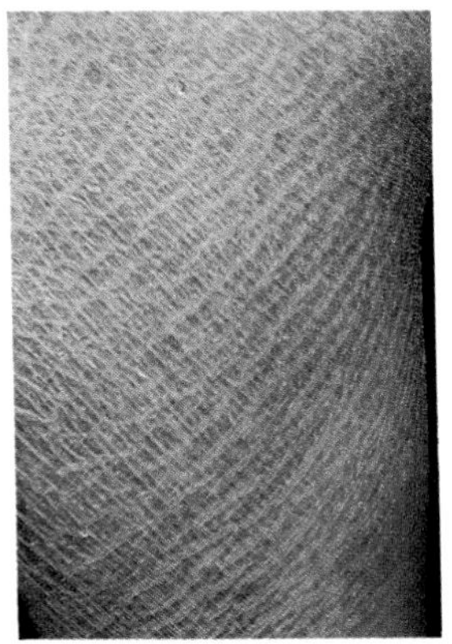

15

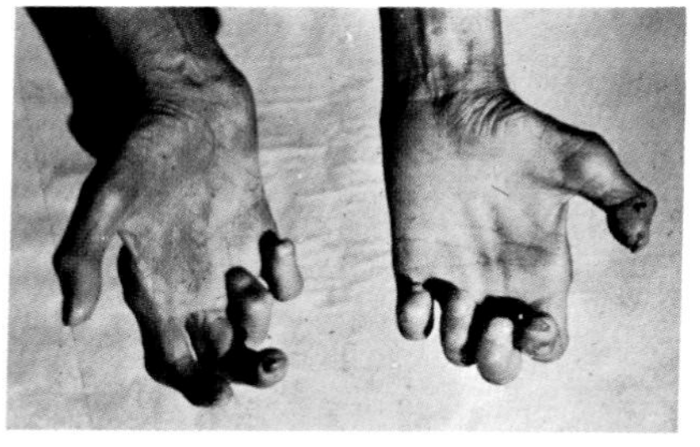

16

Plate 16 Intrinsic muscle wasting due to ulnar and median nerve fibrosis in long-standing lepromatous leprosy. The hands are insensitive. The patient is attempting to extend his fingers.

Plate 17 Type 1 reaction in borderline leprosy. The desquamation is a sign that the reaction is subsiding.

Plate 18 More severe form of Type 2 reaction showing necrotic ENL lesions.

Plate 19 Erythema nodosum leprosum (ENL) in Type 2 reaction.

Plate 20 Eschars in Lucio phenomenon. Note ulceration where one had been removed. Similar lesions were present on buttocks and legs.

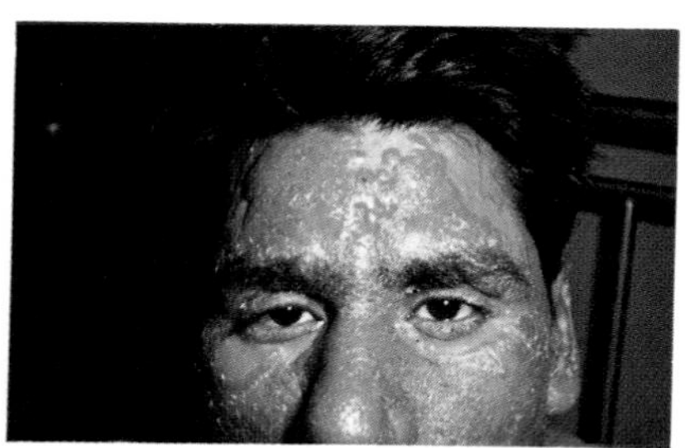

17

19

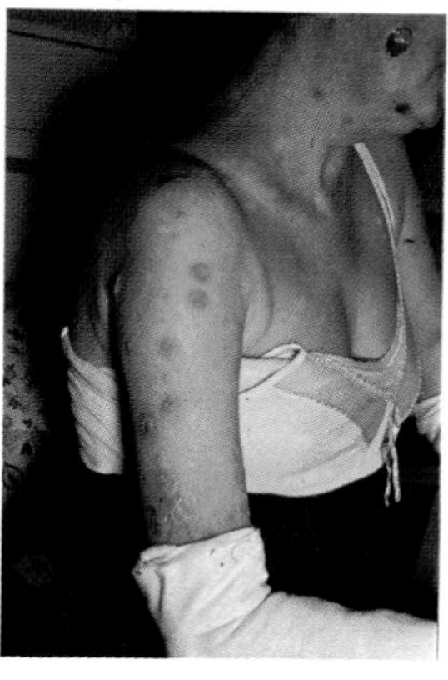

18

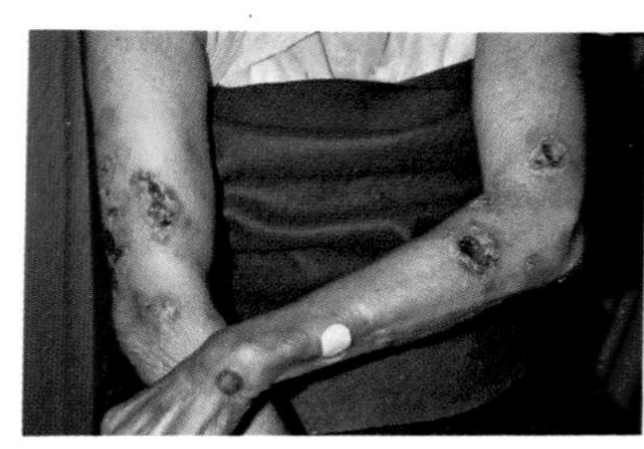

20

skin of patients whose disease is relapsing either because they have stopped treatment or because *M. leprae* has become drug-resistant. Less commonly, a few such nodules may be seen in non-relapsing cases of lepromatous leprosy when first examined.

Although some authors have stressed that these histoid nodules contain elongated or spindle-shaped histiocytes and that the bacilli within them are longer than normal, others have found little to differentiate them histologically and bacteriologically from hyperactive lepromatous nodules. Four papers are recommended for further reading (see references 48, 49, 50 and 51).

Lucio leprosy

This term applies to the diffuse non-nodular type of leprosy described by Lucio and Alvarado in Mexico in 1852 and later by Latapi and Zamora in 1948.[52] Diagnosis is easily overlooked unless note is taken of the shiny thickened skin, the loss of body hair, including eyebrows and eyelashes (but not scalp hair), the puffy hands, and the widespread sensory loss due to involvement of dermal nerves, since nodules and other types of skin lesions are absent. Eyes have a shiny appearance but are free from keratitis or iritis and thickening of upper eyelids gives the patient a sleepy or melancholy look. As in LL, a mild-moderate normochromic and normocytic anaemia is the rule, chronic oedema and chronic ulceration of both legs may develop, ulceration of nasal mucosa may cause nasal symptoms and epistaxis, laryngeal involvement may cause hoarse voice and ichthyosis is a late development. However, unlike LL there are no skin lesions, motor palsies and finger contractions are absent, and the eyes are not damaged.

The patients develop a peculiar form of lepra reaction known as 'Lucio's phenomenon' (see Chapter 6, p. 90). Frenken[30] has translated the original paper by Lucio and Alvarado and has shown that this diffuse type of leprosy is not confined to Mexico as was at one time thought. The fact that the diagnosis is easy to overlook before lepra reaction occurs has been stressed by Donner and Shively,[53] although diagnosis is not difficult once the condition is suspected as skin smears or biopsies from any part of the skin are full of leprosy bacilli. It is easy to see how a wrong diagnosis of myxoedema could be made, bearing in mind the facial appearance, hoarse voice, oedematous legs, and anaemia, and in regions of the world where leprosy is endemic a diagnosis of myxoedema should never be made before examining skin smears for leprosy bacilli.

Tuberculoid leprosy

In contrast to the lepromatous type, the patient with tuberculoid leprosy is likely to report early for medical examination. Looked at purely from the public health viewpoint this is unfortunate, for the patient is non-infectious (i.e. a 'closed' case) whereas the patient with lepromatous leprosy is infectious (i.e. an 'open' case). However, for the patient with tuberculoid leprosy it is fortunate that he has signs and symptoms which take him to the doctor in good time; his symptoms may be neural or dermal, or both. *Neural* symptoms consist of pain, loss of feeling, tinglings and muscle weakness or paralysis. Any of these may occur singly or in combination. A patient was referred to one of the authors because of weakness in fourth and fifth fingers of one hand, and on examination the ulnar nerve on that side was thickened, as was the radial nerve on the lateral border of the wrist. A biopsy of the radial nerve where it was most thickened (the nerve being purely sensory at this site) revealed a tuberculoid histology when the nerve was sectioned, thus establishing the diagnosis of pure neural tuberculoid leprosy. There were no skin lesions. Sensory loss was present.

Another patient reported with a dropped foot; palpation of the lateral popliteal nerve and the superficial peroneal nerve on that side showed thickening, and a biopsy of a thickened branch of the superficial peroneal nerve on the dorsum of the foot confirmed the diagnosis of pure neural tuberculoid leprosy. Diagnosis is easier if a skin lesion appears soon after onset of neural symptoms. A good example of this was the patient who developed pains in one side of the face (5th cranial nerve); his doctor sent him to the dentist but his teeth were found to be healthy. After a week or two he developed facial weakness on that side (7th cranial nerve), and it was only when a red, raised lesion (a plaque) appeared on that same side of his face that the diagnosis of tuberculoid leprosy was considered. Sometimes a skin lesion appears in the absence of neural symptoms. The fact that it is easy to see because it is erythematous or coppery, raised above the general level of the skin, and has well defined edges, means that a doctor's opinion is sought, particularly as the patient may have noticed that the lesion felt numb when touched (i.e. was anaesthetic).

For example, a schoolgirl saw an erythematous plaque on one

arm and reported for medical examination; the plaque was found to be anaesthetic and the ulnar nerve on that side was thickened. A biopsy of the plaque confirmed the diagnosis of tuberculoid leprosy.

A *dermal* lesion of tuberculoid leprosy is usually single, but there may be two or even three. It takes the form of a plaque which may be anywhere on the skin apart from the warmer areas such as the hairy scalp, axillae, groins and perineum. It is erythematous on a light skin, erythematous or coppery on a dark skin, and has a dry surface which is often irregular and sometimes scaly (Plate 5), with raised and well-defined edges and a tendency to central flattening. Hair growth is deficient or absent over the lesion, and sensation is blunted (touch, temperature and pain), but it should be noted that it may be difficult or even impossible to demonstrate impaired sensation in a lesion on the face because of the generous supply of sensory nerves.

Another difficulty may arise if the clinician, testing a lesion for sensory loss, relies solely on a wisp of cotton wool, since light touch sensation is likely to be lost in all those skin diseases in which there is epidermal thickening. A pin is more reliable.

Less commonly the lesion is a macule (level with the surrounding skin), erythematous in light skins and hypopigmented (never *de*pigmented) in dark skins, with sometimes a coppery or orange tint. Such macules are well demarcated and have a dry, hairless and insensitive surface. A thickened nerve is usually palpable in the vicinity of a tuberculoid lesion, whether it be a plaque or a macule, e.g. ulnar nerve if the lesion is near the elbow, radial cutaneous nerve if near the wrist, etc., or a thickened nerve may be felt leaving (or entering), the lesion; such a sensory nerve will be missed by the examiner if he does not run his finger lightly all the way around the edge of the lesion, for the thickened nerve is detected by feeling and not by sight. Nerve thickening may be smooth or irregular, and rarely a cystic swelling may be seen and felt in relation to a nerve – a cold abscess of nerve. Even more rare is calcification in a nerve (Fig. 2.11). The authors have encountered it in only two patients, both suffering from pure neural tuberculoid leprosy and both giving a past history of nerve abscess; one ulnar nerve was affected in both cases.

In addition to testing tuberculoid lesions for sensory loss, a

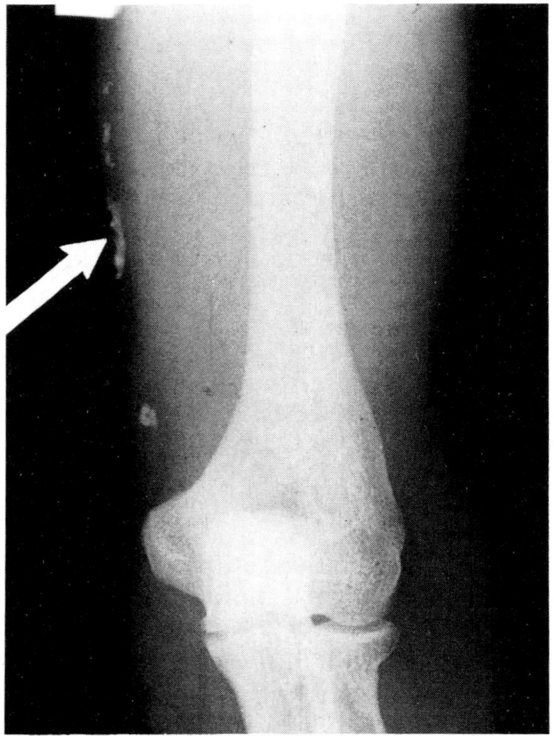

Fig. 2.11 Calcification in an ulnar nerve in tuberculoid leprosy (a pure neural case).

sweating test can demonstrate anhidrosis and a histamine test on a hypopigmented lesion shows absence of flare (Chapter 4). These tests confirm that dermal nerves are damaged. Skin smears and nasal scrapings (Chapter 4) are negative.

Borderline leprosy

As can be seen in Fig. 2.4, this type of leprosy occurs in those whose degree of resistance lies somewhere in the spectrum between lepromatous and tuberculoid, and therefore the number of lesions and their clinical features vary according to the position in the spectrum. It is not generally appreciated that borderline leprosy is the most common type of leprosy to be encountered if we take a global view, and failure to appreciate this fact is due to

Type	Skin and nerve changes	Bacteriology	Histology (dermis)	Immunology
T	A single macule or plaque (two or three at most), anaesthetic, anhidrotic, hairless, with well-defined edges. Early nerve thickening (one or two nerves only).	AFB absent in skin lesions and nasal mucosa.	Foci of lymphocytes, epithelioid cells and giant cells invading papillary zone and sometimes eroding epidermis. Cutaneous nerves, if not destroyed, are greatly swollen by epithelioid cell granuloma; they may caseate.	Lepromin reaction strongly positive.
B	Macules, plaques, annular lesions and punched-out lesions distributed asymmetrically. Macules have well-defined edges; plaques have edges which are vague in parts and there is little central flattening; annular and punched-out lesions are classical. All show some degree of sensory loss; they are too numerous and not dry enough for TT, they are too large, too few, and not shiny enough for LL. On the TT side of the spectrum lesions are less numerous, are drier and more anaesthetic; on the LL side they are more numerous, more shiny, and less anaesthetic. Early nerve thickening (several nerves).	In BL lesions AFB are numerous but globi unusual, AFB moderate in BB and few or absent in BT. AFB scanty in uninvolved skin and nasal mucosa in BL, absent in BB and BT.	In BL there is a granuloma composed of macrophages with lymphocytes in dense clumps or sheets. In BB there is a diffuse epithelioid cell granuloma. In BT there is a tuberculoid reaction more diffuse than in TT. In all three there is a free subepidermal zone, and cutaneous nerves contain cellular infiltrate	Lepromin reaction negative in BL and BB, weakly or moderately positive in BT.
L	In LLp and LLs there are numerous macules, papules and nodules, distributed bilaterally and symmetrically, having normal sensation and hair growth. Lesions are shiny and macules have vague edges. Nerve thickening in late stages, but in LLs there is evidence of a previous borderline phase in the form of thickened nerves and some typical borderline lesions.	AFB numerous in lesions and nasal mucosa. Globi usual. AFB numerous in clinically uninvolved skin, especially fingers.	Thinned epidermis and flattened rete ridge. Diffuse leproma of foamy macrophages with few lymphocytes and plasma cells. Comparing LLs with LLp, foamy change is decreased or absent, lymphocytes are increased, and cutaneous nerves may show slight cellular infiltrate.	Lepromin reaction negative.
I	Entirely macular. Usually a single macule with fairly well-defined edges, slight or absent sensory loss, and depressed histamine flare.	AFB absent (rarely one bacillus in a cutaneous nerve).	Non-specific cellular reaction with tendency to surround skin appendages.	Lepromin reaction unpredictable.

AFB = Acid-fast bacilli; B = Borderline; BB = Mid-borderline; BL = Borderline lepromatous; BT = Borderline tuberculoid; I = Indeterminate; L (LL) = Lepromatous; LLp = Polar lepromatous; LLs = Supolar lepromatous.

(Reproduced from Jopling W. H., Harman R. R. M. (1986). Leprosy. In *Textbook of Dermatology*, 4th edn. Oxford: Blackwell Scientific Publications.)

The Indian classification

This describes six forms of leprosy:[62] Lepromatous (L); Tuberculoid (T); Maculoanaesthetic (MA); Polyneuritic (pure neural) (P); Borderline (B) and Indeterminate (I). The definitions of L, T, and I do not depart from those generally accepted worldwide. Compared with the Ridley–Jopling classification (see Table 2.1, p. 43) the following can be noted: the Indian classification gives only one borderline group but accepts that there are, 'great morphological variations within the group', and describes the lepromin reaction as 'variable, never strongly positive'. Histology does not recognise distinctive subgroups, but accepts a clear subepidermal zone. In the MA group, skin lesions are described as macular, with well-defined edges and definite anaesthesia, absent bacilli in skin smears and a lepromin reaction which is moderately or strongly positive. This would include BT and TT. The indeterminate form is not included in the Ridley–Jopling classification. As regards P, there is no deviation from the pure neural leprosy included within the TT–LL spectrum of Ridley–Jopling classification (see p. 42).

Reasons for classification in leprosy

What are the reasons for classification in leprosy? First, a correct classification will give essential information on whether a patient is infectious or not, on the prognosis, on the choice of chemotherapy and the length of treatment, and on the likelihood of complications, such as lepra reaction. Second, a classification which is widely known and applied enables clinicians to communicate intelligently with others. Third, when patients are selected for research projects, it is essential that their leprosy is accurately classified if faulty conclusions are to be avoided (Tables 2.1 and 2.3).

REFERENCES

1 Fisher C. A., Barksdale L. (1971). Elimination of the acid-fastness but not the gram positivity of leprosy bacilli after extraction with pyridine. *Journal of Bacteriology*; **106**: 707–8.

2 Dutta A. K., Katoch V. M., Sharma V. D., Katoch K. (1984). Effect of pyridine extraction on the acid-fastness of *M. leprae*:

its possible mechanism. Abstract IV/219(A) in XII *International Leprosy Congress Abstracts*.
3 Draper P. (1986). Structure of *Mycobacterium leprae*. *Leprosy Review* (Suppl. 2); **57**: 15–20.
4 Ridley D. S. (1958). Therapeutic trials in leprosy using serial biopsies. *Leprosy Review*; **29**: 45–52.
5 Waters M. F. R., Rees R. J. W. (1962). Changes in the morphology of *Mycobacterium leprae* in patients under treatment. *International Journal of Leprosy*; **30**: 266–77.
6 Hansen G. A., Looft C. (1895). *Leprosy: in its clinical and pathological aspects*. Reprinted by John Wright, Bristol, 1973.
7 Ridley D. S. (1971). The SFG (solid, fragmented, granular) index for bacterial morphology. *Leprosy Review*; **42**: 96–7.
8 Ridley D. S. (1955). The bacteriological interpretations of skin smears and biopsies in leprosy. *Transactions of the Royal Society of Tropical Medicine & Hygiene*; **49**: 449–52.
9 Ridley D. S. (1958). Therapeutic trials in leprosy using serial biopsies. *Leprosy Review*; **29**: 45–52.
10 Ridley D. S. (1967). A logarithmic index of bacilli in biopsies. *International Journal of Leprosy*; **35**: 187–93.
11 Hansen G. A. (1874). Spedalskhedens arsager. *Norsk Magazin for Laegervidenskaben*; **4**: 76–9. Translated by Pallamary P. (1955). Causes of leprosy. *International Journal of Leprosy*; **23**: 307–9.
12 Shepard C. C. (1960). The experimental disease that follows the injection of human leprosy bacilli into the foot-pads of mice. *Journal of Experimental Medicine*; **112**: 445–54.
13 Rees R. J. W. (1966). Enhanced susceptibility of thymectomised and irradiated mice to infection with *Mycobacterium leprae*. *Nature*; **211**: 657–8.
14 Godal T., Negassi K. (1973). Subclinical infection in leprosy. *British Medical Journal*; **3**: 557–9.
15 Weddell G., Palmer E., Rees R. J. W., Jamison D. G. (1963). In *The Pathogenesis of Leprosy* (Wolstenholme G. E. W., O'Conor M., eds) p. 3115. London: J. & A. Churchill Limited.
16 Pearson J. M. H., Ross W. F. (1975). Nerve involvement in leprosy – pathology, differential diagnosis and principles of management. *Leprosy Review*; **46**: 199–212.
17 Brand P. W. (1959). Temperature variation and leprosy deformity. *International Journal of Leprosy*: **27**: 1–7.

18 Jopling W. H., Morgan-Hughes J. A. (1965). Pure neural tuberculoid leprosy. *British Medical Journal*; **2**: 799–800.
19 Ridley D. S. (1974). Histological classification and the immunological spectrum of leprosy. *Bulletin of the World Health Organization*; **51**: 451–65.
20 Jopling W. H. (1956). Borderline (dimorphous) leprosy maintaining a polyneuritic form for eight years: a case report. *Transactions of the Royal Society of Tropical Medicine & Hygiene*; **50**: 478–80.
21 Hanks J. H. (1945). A note on the number of leprosy bacilli which may occur in leprous nodules. *International Journal of Leprosy*; **13**: 25–6.
22 Job C. K., Desikan K. V. (1968). Pathologic changes and their distribution in peripheral nerves in lepromatous leprosy. *International Journal of Leprosy*; **36**: 257–70.
23 Gupta M., Bhargava M., Kumar S., Mittal M. M. (1975). Platelet function in leprosy. *International Journal of Leprosy*; **43**: 327–32.
24 Cole F. S., Brusch J. L., Talarico L. (1979). A circulating anticoagulant in lepromatous leprosy. *International Journal of Leprosy*; **47**: 121–5.
25 Ridley D. S., Jopling W. H. (1966). Classification of leprosy according to immunity. *International Journal of Leprosy*; **34**: 255–73.
26 Rees R. J. W. (1965). Recent bacteriologic, immunologic and pathologic studies on experimental human leprosy in the mouse foot pad. *International Journal of Leprosy*; **33**: 646–55.
27 Ridley D. S. (1986). The classification of Hansen's Disease. The *STAR*; **45**: 8–10.
28 McDougall A. C., Archibald G. C. (1977). Lepromatous leprosy presenting with swelling of legs. *British Medical Journal*; **1**: 23–4.
29 Dutta A. K., Mandal S. B., Jopling W. H. (1983). Surface temperature of bald and hairy scalp in reference to leprosy affection. *Indian Journal of Dermatology*; **28**: 1–5.
30 Frenken J. H. (1963). *Diffuse leprosy of Lucio and Latapi*. Detroit: Blaine Ethridge.
31 Møller-Christensen V. (1961). *Bone Changes of Leprosy*. Bristol: John Wright.
32 Møller-Christensen V. (1974). Changes in the anterior nasal

spine and the alveolar process of the maxillae in leprosy: a clinical examination. *International Journal of Leprosy*; **42**: 431–5.

33 Chaco J., Magora A., Zauberman H., Landau Y. (1968). An electromyographic study of lagophthalmos in leprosy. *International Journal of Leprosy*; **36**: 288–95.

34 Jopling W. H. (1978). Vitiligo and leprosy. *Leprosy Review*; **49**: 88.

35 Barton R. P. E. (1974). Olfaction in leprosy. *Journal of Laryngology and Otology*; **88**: 355–61.

36 Barton R. P. E. (1974). A clinical study of the nose in lepromatous leprosy. *Leprosy Review*; **45**: 135–44.

37 Girdhar B. K., Desikan K. V. (1979). A clinical study of the mouth in untreated lepromatous patients. *Leprosy Review*; **50**: 25–35.

38 Hobbs H. E., Choyce D. P. (1971). The blinding lesions of leprosy. *Leprosy Review*; **42**: 131–7.

39 ffytche T. J. (1981). The eye and leprosy. *Leprosy Review*; **52**: 111–19.

40 Warren G. (1972). The management of tarsal bone disintegration. *Leprosy Review*; **43**: 137–47.

41 Sharma S. C., Kumar B., Dhall K., Kaur S., Malhotra S., Aikat M. (1981). Leprosy and female reproductive organs. *International Journal of Leprosy*; **49**: 177–9.

42 Johny K. V., Karat A. B. A., Rao P. S. S., Date A. (1975). Glomerulonephritis in leprosy – a percutaneous renal biopsy study. *Leprosy Review*; **46**: 29–37.

43 Desikan K. V., Job C. K. (1968). A review of postmortem findings in 37 cases of leprosy. *International Journal of Leprosy*; **36**: 32–44.

44 Zemer D., Pras M., Sohar E., Modan M., Cabil S., Gafni J. (1986). Colchicine in the prevention and treatment of the amyloidosis of familial Mediterranean fever. *New England Journal of Medicine*; **314**: 1001–5.

45 Jopling W. H., Mehta H. D. (1972). A case of leprous nodular interstitial myositis. *Leprosy Review*; **43**: 39–43.

46 Shwe T., Thein M., Myint S. (1975). Prevalence of pulmonary tuberculosis in patients with leprosy. *Burma Medical Journal*; **21**: 39–44.

47 Parikh A. A., Shah B. H. (1986). Tetanus in a case of lepromatous leprosy. *Indian Journal of Leprosy*; **58**: 628–9.

48 Wade H. W. (1963). The histoid variety of lepromatous leprosy. *International Journal of Leprosy*; **31**: 129–42.

49 Rodriguez J. N. (1969). The histoid leproma: its characteristics and significance. *International Journal of Leprosy*; **37**: 1–21.

50 Bhutani L. K., Bedi T. R., Malhotra Y. K., Kandhari K. C., Deo M. G. (1974). Histoid leprosy in North India. *International Journal of Leprosy*; **42**: 174–81.

51 Ridley M. J., Ridley D. S. (1980). Histoid leprosy. An ultrastructural observation. *International Journal of Leprosy*; **48**: 135–9.

52 Latapi F., Zamora A. C. (1948). The 'spotted' leprosy of Lucio (la lepra 'manchada' de Lucio): an introduction to its clinical and histological study. *International Journal of Leprosy*; **16**: 421–30.

53 Donner R. S., Shively J. A. (1967). The 'Lucio phenomenon' in diffuse leprosy. *Annals of Internal Medicine*; **67**: 831–6.

54 Leiker D. L. (1964). Low-resistant tuberculoid leprosy. *International Journal of Leprosy*; **32**: 359–67.

55 Price J. E. (1982). BCG vaccination in leprosy. *International Journal of Leprosy*; **50**: 205–12.

56 Duncan M. E., Melsom R., Pearson J. M. H., Ridley D. S. (1981). The association of pregnancy and leprosy. I. New cases, relapse of cured patients and deterioration in patients on treatment during pregnancy and lactation – results of a prospective study of 154 pregnancies in 147 Ethiopian women. *Leprosy Review*; **52**: 245–62.

57 Duncan M. E., Pearson J. M. H., Ridley D. S., Melsom R., Bjune G. (1982). Pregnancy and leprosy: the consequences of alterations of cell-mediated and humoral immunity during pregnancy and lactation. *International Journal of Leprosy*; **50**: 425–35.

58 Duncan M. E., Pearson J. M. H. (1982). Neuritis in pregnancy and lactation. *International Journal of Leprosy*; **50**: 31–8.

59 Duncan M. E. (1980). Babies of mothers with leprosy have small placentae, low birth weights and grow slowly. *British Journal of Obstetrics & Gynaecology*; **87**: 471–9.

60 Ridley D. S., Waters M. F. R. (1969). Significance of variations within the lepromatous group. *Leprosy Review*; **40**: 143–52.

61 Ridley D. S. (1982). The pathogenesis and classification of polar tuberculoid leprosy. *Leprosy Review*; **53**: 19–26.
62 Dharmendra (1978). *Leprosy*, Vol. 1. Bombay: Kothari Medical Publishing House.

3 The Lepromin Test

Although this is a non-specific test which is positive in the majority of healthy adults in regions where leprosy is non-endemic, and cannot be used as a diagnostic test, it is of great value in classifying a case of leprosy once the diagnosis has been made. It is a delayed-type hypersensitivity reaction to *M. leprae* or its antigens, and is a guide to the resistance of the patient. One type of lepromin, known as Mitsuda lepromin (integral lepromin of Mitsuda–Wade–Hayashi), is an autoclaved suspension of tissue derived from experimentally infected armadillos (lepromin A), which has replaced Mitsuda lepromin derived from human tissue (lepromin H), and is standardised. Details of its manufacture will be found in the *Bulletin of the WHO*, Vol. 57(6), 1979. It contains 1.6×10^8 bacilli (160 million) per ml,[1] has a shelf life of 2 years, and the bottle must be shaken vigorously before use. It is named after the Japanese leprologist who as long ago as 1916 introduced a skin test, using material from leprosy nodules, on the strength of which he classified his patients as 'neuromacular' if a positive reaction was obtained, and as 'nodular' if the reaction was negative.[2]

MITSUDA REACTION

An injection of 0.1 ml is given intradermally using the smallest needle obtainable and a Mantoux syringe (the authors use a disposable needle size 26G × $^3/_8$) and the size of the weal should measure 8–10 mm in diameter. The size should be recorded. A suitable site for the injection is the flexor surface of the left forearm 2–3 cm below the elbow crease. If this site is always used as a routine there will be no likelihood of confusion when the result of the test is read after 4–5 weeks, particularly if other skin tests may have been carried out in the interim and, more especially, if the person who reads the test is not the one who injected the lepromin. The Mitsuda reaction can be described as follows:

Negative (−)	Nothing to see or feel
Doubtful (±)	A papule 3 mm or less in diameter
One-plus positive (+)	An erythematous papule 4–7 mm in diameter without ulceration
Two-plus positive (++)	An erythematous papule larger than 7 mm and up to 10 mm in diameter without ulceration
Three-plus positive (+++)	An erythematous nodule larger than 10 mm, or one of any size with ulceration

This system has been recommended by the Expert Committee on Leprosy in the WHO Technical Report Series, No. 71 (1953) for the late reaction at 4 weeks. One of the authors (WHJ) accepts 3–6 mm as a one-plus (+) reaction, and 7–10 mm as a two-plus (++) reaction in the absence of ulceration.

The WHO recommends that the letter 'U' should be added to the reading of the size of the reaction if ulceration is present. It also recommends that the reaction should be recorded at 4 weeks when testing leprosy patients and contacts. The solution should be shaken before use.

In some Mitsuda-positive persons an early reaction can be seen at 48 hours and takes the form of erythema and induration; it is known as a Fernandez reaction and is generally considered to be a manifestation of delayed hypersensitivity (Chapter 5) to bacillary antigen, in contrast to the Mitsuda reaction at 4 weeks which is a more reliable index of cell-mediated immunity. As the early reaction is not always present when the Mitsuda reaction is positive, and as it may be vague and difficult to interpret, most clinicians ignore it and concentrate on the late reading. The Fernandez reaction is best seen when using Dharmendra's lepromin (see below) but, when testing contacts of leprosy patients or children who have indeterminate leprosy, the Mitsuda reaction is a better guide as to the type of leprosy which may ensue. The Mitsuda reaction is (+++) in TT, (++) in BT nearer the tuberculoid end of the spectrum, (+) in BT nearer the middle of the spectrum, and negative in BB, BL and LL (see Fig. 2.12).

FERNANDEZ REACTION

In 1941 and 1942 Dharmendra[2,3,4] published his researches on the production of a bacillary type of lepromin by separating bacilli from human tissue, and on extracting the soluble protein fraction from leprosy bacilli. He concluded that the early reaction at 48 hours seen when using bacillary lepromin was due to the protein fraction released from bacilli broken in the process of preparing the antigen, and the late reaction at 4 weeks was due to the slow release of the same fraction from the originally intact bacilli. This type of lepromin has been in use ever since, chiefly in India, and is known as Dharmendra lepromin. It is a purified chloroform-ether-extracted suspension of *M. leprae* and is practically devoid of human tissue; 0.1 ml is injected intradermally and the result is seen at 48 hours. If positive it resembles a positive Mantoux (tuberculin) reaction, and one looks for (and measures) an area of erythema and induration. The reaction derives its name from the Argentinian leprologist, J. M. M. Fernandez, who was one of the pioneers in the production of a bacillary lepromin. There is also a late reading at 4 weeks, a papulonodule if the reaction is positive, but this is smaller than the Mitsuda reaction and does not ulcerate. In other words, both Mitsuda and Dharmendra lepromin produce an early and a late reaction, the early one being most readily seen with Dharmendra lepromin and the late one being most prominent with Mitsuda lepromin.

The Fernandez reaction is recorded as follows:

Negative (−)	Nothing to see, or erythema without induration, or erythema and induration less than 5 mm in diameter
Weakly positive (+)	Erythema and induration 5–10 mm in diameter
Moderately positive (++)	Erythema and induration 11–15 mm in diameter
Strongly positive (+++)	Erythema and induration 16 mm or more in diameter

Note: The fleeting reactions which may occur before 48 hours are of very doubtful value. The above readings are really averages since the reaction is sometimes irregular rather than round, in which case one measures the largest and smallest diameters and the mean of the two readings is taken.

NEWER SKIN TEST MATERIAL WITH IMPROVED SPECIFICITY FOR *M. LEPRAE*

As previously mentioned, the lepromin test, although valuable in classification of known leprosy patients, is a non-specific test, often being positive in persons who have never had contact with *M. leprae*. Research is proceeding in the production and testing of purified protein derivatives (PPDs) of *M. leprae*, encouraged by the WHO programme of research on immunity of leprosy (IMM-LEP), in the hope that they will prove more specific for leprosy. One which is under investigation is 'leprosin' which is prepared from *M. leprae* by ultrasonication, ultracentrifugation and sterile filtration. But research on the identification of *M. leprae* antigens, aided by the use of monoclonal antibodies in identifying antigens which are functionally important (see Chapter 5), is likely to produce a breakthrough. In this way, the WHO is encouraging the completion of the early researches of Dharmendra, and this important work has been made possible by the large supplies of *M. leprae* which can now be produced by infected armadillos. Having to rely on human resources for *M. leprae* has been the great stumbling block in the past.

REFERENCES

1 WHO Expert Committee on Leprosy (1970). 4th Report. *Technical Report Series No. 459*. Geneva: WHO.
2 Dharmendra (1942). The immunological skin tests in leprosy. Part 1: The isolation of a protein antigen of *Mycobacterium leprae*. *Indian Journal of Medical Research*; **30**: 1–7.
3 Dharmendra (1941). Studies of the lepromin test. (5) The active principle of lepromin is a protein antigen of the bacillus. *Leprosy in India*; **13**: 89–103.
4 Dharmendra (1942). Studies of the lepromin test. (9) A bacillus antigen standardised by weight. *Leprosy in India*; **14**: 122–9.

4 Diagnostic Tests

SKIN SMEARS

The lesion is cleaned with ether and a portion of it is gripped between thumb and forefinger of the left hand to drive out the blood. With a small-bladed scalpel (e.g. size 15 Bard Parker blade) an incision is made between the fingers of the left hand about 5 mm long and 3 mm deep, pressure of the fingers being maintained. The blade is then turned at right angles to the cut and the wound is scraped several times in the same direction so that tissue fluid and pulp (not blood) collects on one side of the blade; this is gently smeared on a glass slide. The smear is fixed over a flame before being sent for staining. Two or more smears can be made on one slide, each being numbered with a marking pencil, and a total of six or eight should be made. The sites of the smears are recorded, so that the same sites can be used for successive sets of smears during the course of treatment. Slides with smears on them should not be exposed to sunlight, dust, extremes of temperature and humidity, since these factors may interfere with the capacity of bacilli to take up carbol fuchsin in the Ziehl–Neelsen staining method. Another factor interfering with good staining is long storage of fixed slides.[1] Furthermore, smears which are left on a shelf or office desk overnight appeal to the voracious appetite of cockroaches, and this may lead to the dissemination of viable leprosy bacilli, for it has recently been shown that the oriental cockroach ingesting sputum smears is able to excrete viable tubercle bacilli.[2] Faulty results will be obtained if the incision is not sufficient to include the deepest portion of the dermis, for it is useless to examine a smear consisting of epidermal cells. Observations at the Hospital for Tropical Diseases, London, have shown that in long-treated lepromatous patients the skin sites where bacilli are most frequently detected, whether granular or solid-staining, are the dorsa of fingers,[3] and smears from fingers give the earliest indication of impending relapse.[4] In a follow-up of 116 multibacillary patients who had received multidrug therapy in the Malta-Project, skin smears from six sites (two from fingers) revealed scanty solid-staining bacilli in 10 patients; one or other finger was positive for 'solids' in 8 of these 10 patients, but in 7 of them the fingers were the *only* positive sites.[5] See p. 96 for the recording of smears.

WHO guidelines for making smears and avoiding the risk of AIDS

In order to eliminate any risk of transmitting the human immunodeficiency virus (HIV) either from patient-to-patient or patient-to-health worker, when making skin smears, the WHO has published guidelines, and these will be found in *Leprosy Review* (September 1987; **58**: 207).

Guide to making and staining of smears

A booklet entitled *Technical Guide for Smear Examination for Leprosy* by D. L. Leiker and A. C. McDougall (1983), is published by the Leprosy Documentation Service (INFOLEP). Requests for copies should be addressed to the German Leprosy Relief Association, Postfach 348, D-8700, Würzburg, West Germany.

NASAL SCRAPINGS

These are not necessary as a routine, and there are three situations in which they can be positively misleading:

1. When taken in order to establish a diagnosis they can be misleading as more leprosy patients have negative nasal scrapings than negative skin smears. Probably 75% of all leprosy patients have negative nasal scrapings at the time of diagnosis.
2. Scanty acid-fast bacilli are sometimes found in healthy noses and may cause diagnostic confusion. However, the experienced bacteriologist is not likely to be misled by the presence of a few AFB as he knows that when nasal scrapings are positive in leprosy the bacilli are present in large numbers, including many globi.

3 Not only does the inexperienced clinician find nasal scrapings difficult to make, especially as it is unlikely that he will possess a suitable instrument, but he is likely to select the anterior portion of the nasal septum; this is the least likely site in the nose to yield positive results.

Although routine nasal scrapings are not recommended, they are of great importance if it is a question of deciding if a leprosy patient is infectious or not. They are always positive in untreated lepromatous leprosy but are negative in most cases of BL and in all cases of BB, BT and TT. Furthermore, they disappear more rapidly from the nose, as a result of chemotherapy, than they do from skin lesions.

Method

Although a piece of bicycle spoke is usually recommended, the ideal instrument is the small round curette made by Downs Surgical Limited (catalogue number HV–210–01–D). There are three sizes, and the most practical sizes for the purpose are 1 and 2 (2 being a little larger than 1). With the aid of a torch and nasal speculum, scrapings should be taken from the anterior part of the inferior turbinates,[6] where they jut out into the nasal cavity, one scraping from each side. The material in the curette, which usually is slightly bloodstained, is picked up with the tip of a scalpel blade and smeared onto a glass slide. Nasal secretions collected by nose blowing (nose-blows) provide an alternative means of assessing a patient's infectivity. Pedley[7] found that the majority of his untreated lepromatous patients had leprosy bacilli in their nasal discharge, often in very great numbers, but only 1 out of 41 of his most active borderline patients had positive nasal mucus. In a new lepromatous patient nasal scrapings and nose-blows will have a higher percentage of solid-staining (viable) bacilli than will be found in skin smears.

Smears of nasal secretions (nose-blows) are best prepared from early morning nose-blows. The patient blows his nose thoroughly into a clean, dry, small sheet of plastic film. Either the smear may be made beside the patient, or the plastic may be folded, labelled, and sent to the laboratory in a sterile container. To make the smear, an aliquot of the nasal discharge is transferred to a labelled glass microscope slide, and spread as evenly as possible. If the discharge consists of both watery and opaque material, the latter should be selected. A platinum loop is not rigid enough to spread thick nasal discharge, especially if crusts are present. It is better to use a small cotton-wool swab, slightly moistened in normal saline and held by forceps. (These directions are taken from *Laboratory Techniques for Leprosy*. (1987). Geneva: WHO.)

SKIN BIOPSY

This is helpful in diagnosis and valuable for correct classification. The lesion is cleaned with ether and covered with a sterile towel which has a small square cut out of the centre. One millilitre of 1% or 2% lignocaine is drawn up into a syringe and mixed with Hyalase (spreading factor).

After injecting a small quantity intradermally the needle is inserted into the centre of the anaesthetised area of skin and driven downwards in stages, injecting local anaesthetic at each stage until the needle can go no further. A Schick needle (13 mm) is ideal for this purpose as its full length gives adequate anaesthesia for a full-depth biopsy (*a biopsy in leprosy must include the full depth of the dermis together with a portion of subcutaneous fat*). A scalpel can be used for removing the piece of skin, but the authors' preference is for a skin biopsy punch which can be inserted with a rotary action. A punch with a cutting edge of 5 mm diameter is suitable and the wound will require only one stitch. A suitable metal punch is the Hayes Martin skin punch (obtainable from Chas. F. Thackray Ltd, PO Box 171, Leeds LS1 1RQ. Quote No. 66–3859, and request cutting edge diameter (3, 4, or 5 mm)) but the authors prefer disposable punches obtained from Stiefel Laboratories (UK) Ltd, Wellcroft Road, Slough, England. These can also be obtained from their French or German branches; one has to choose between a cutting edge diameter of 4 mm or of 6 mm, as there is no intermediate size available. It should be noted that in biopsy work there is no need to include normal skin at the edge of the lesion. A dressing strip is applied and the patient is advised to keep it dry. The stitch is removed after 1 week. The operator must take the greatest care not to damage the biopsy material when it is picked up with dissecting forceps, and toothed forceps must *never* be used.

Histopathology service

Where there is a need for such a service, specimens can be sent to Dr S. B. Lucas, Department of Morbid Anatomy, School of Medicine, University College Hospital, University Street, London WC1. A short account of the clinical findings in each case should be included. In the case of a skin biopsy, record the site of the biopsy, and for choice of fixative solution in which to send it, see 'A note on fixative solutions', p. 65. *Leprosy Review* ((1982); **53**: 67–8) gives advice on the transporting of histopathological specimens.

When a biopsy is being sent for a foot pad test, it should be placed in a small sterile bottle without any additive and kept at 4°C until dispatch in a thermos flask containing ice.

NERVE BIOPSY

This is essential in a pure neural example and will show typical tuberculoid or borderline histology as the case may be, together with bacilli in most borderline cases, but nerve biopsy will not be required if a skin lesion is present. A thickened sensory nerve is suitable, such as a supraorbital branch of the 5th cranial nerve (Plate 8), a supraclavicular nerve, the great auricular nerve in the neck, the radial nerve at the wrist, a cutaneous nerve of forearm or thigh, the sural nerve at the back of the leg or at the lateral border of the foot, or a superficial peroneal nerve on the dorsum of the foot (Plate 11). These nerves do not contain motor fibres and therefore there is no risk of motor damage (see Fig 2.5a and b). Pearson[8] favours the radial cutaneous nerve and has described his technique. A generous amount of 2% procaine with added hyaluronidase (Hyalase) is injected *around* the nerve, and after waiting for 5 to 10 minutes a transverse skin crease incision is made at about the level of the styloid process of the radius, and the nerve is separated by blunt dissection. A small nick is made in the nerve, to divide one or two fasciculi, which are then picked up and stripped from the nerve bundle for about 1 cm by careful sharp dissection. If the nerve is much damaged by the leprosy process, and fasciculi are obliterated, a small longitudinal wedge of nerve can be removed. The excised portion is immediately immersed in fixative.

A note on fixative solutions

A fixative is the solution into which the biopsy material is placed, and the choice of fixative is important. If it is defective it may be impossible to cut good sections and stain them properly. For nerve biopsies (to be done by experts only) 10% buffered formalin is quite satisfactory, but for skin, better results can be obtained by using a solution such as 'FMA' fixative (40% formaldehyde 10 ml, mercuric chloride 2 g, glacial acetic acid 3 ml, water to 100 ml).[9] If this is used, the specimen is transferred to 70% alcohol after 2 hours without washing in water; it can be left in the alcohol for an indefinite period. This may be too difficult in remote areas, in which case freshly prepared, buffered 10% formalin may be used.

HISTAMINE TEST

When histamine is injected intradermally into normal skin it causes capillary dilatation, and this can be seen as a bright red flare known as a histamine flare. This effect is not a direct one on capillary walls but is produced by an axon reflex within dermal nerves. Therefore, histamine can be used to test the integrity of dermal nerves, and the degree of damage to these nerves can be gauged by the reduction in size and brightness of the histamine flare. This can be useful in deciding if a hypopigmented macule is due to leprosy.

Method

One drop of histamine acid phosphate (diphosphate) 1 in 1000 (1 mg in 1 ml) is placed on the area of skin to be tested and another on a control site. A superficial prick is made through each drop, and a bright flare will appear if dermal nerves are intact; it will appear within a minute on face or trunk but takes a little longer on a limb. In a leprosy macule the flare is delayed, feeble or entirely absent; it is delayed and feeble in indeterminate and borderline leprosy, and absent in a tuberculoid lesion. If the hypopigmented macule is due to a non-leprosy condition it will give a normal flare, e.g. vitiligo, fungal infection, yaws, etc. The situation is different if the patient complains of an area of skin anaesthesia in the absence of skin lesions, for there is a depression of histamine flare in all types of peripheral neuropathy (including leprosy); for example, the test cannot help in deciding if an areas of sensory loss on the antero-lateral aspect of the thigh is due to meralgia paraesthetica (Bernhardt's syndrome) or to leprous involvement of one or more of the femoral cutaneous nerves (see Fig. 2.5b.). However, it is of great help in ruling out hysteria or an abnormality of brain or spinal cord, for in these conditions a normal flare is obtained. In Lucio leprosy (p. 37) there is depression or absence of flare all over the skin.

SWEATING TEST

This is another method of testing the integrity of dermal nerves. Anhidrosis is characteristic of skin lesions in tuberculoid leprosy, and one method of testing is to inject intradermally 0.2 ml of a 1 in 1000 solution of pilocarpine nitrate into the lesion to be tested, to paint the injection site with tincture of iodine, and then to dust with starch powder.

Quinizarin powder can be used in place of starch, in which case there is no need to paint with iodine. Sweating causes a blue discoloration of the powder, whereas there is no blue colour if sweating is absent due to damage to dermal nerves.

REFERENCES

1 Sayer J., Gent R., Jesudasan K. (1987). Are bacterial counts on slit-skin smears in leprosy affected by preparing slides under field conditions? *Leprosy Review*; **58**: 271–8.
2 Allen B. W. (1987). Excretion of viable tubercle bacilli by *Blatta orientalis* (the oriental cockroach) following ingestion of heat-fixed sputum smears: a laboratory investigation. *Transactions of the Royal Society of Tropical Medicine & Hygiene*; **81**: 98–9.
3 Ridley M. J., Jopling W. H., Ridley D. S. (1976). Acid-fast bacilli in the fingers of long-treated lepromatous patients. *Leprosy Review*; **47**: 93–6.
4 Jopling W. H., Rees R. J. W., Ridley D. S., Ridley M. J., Samuel N. M. (1979). The fingers as sites of leprosy bacilli in pre-relapse patients. *Leprosy Review*; **50**: 289–92.
5 Jopling W. H., Ridley M. J., Bonnici E., Depasquale G. (1984). A follow-up investigation of the Malta-Project. *Leprosy Review*; **55**: 247–53.

6 Barton R. P. E. (1974). A clinical study of the nose in lepromatous leprosy. *Leprosy Review*; **45**: 135–44.
7 Pedley J. C. (1973). The nasal mucus in leprosy. *Leprosy Review*; **44**: 33–5.
8 Pearson J. M. H., Weddell G. (1971). Changes in sensory acuity following radial nerve biopsy in patients with leprosy. *Brain*; **94**: 43–50.
9 Ridley D. S. (1958). Therapeutic trials in leprosy using serial biopsies. *Leprosy Review*; **29**: 45–52.

5 General Principles of Immunology and their Application to the Leprosy Patient

If it could be shown that different types of leprosy are due to peculiarities of the organism infecting individual patients, then leprosy would not be attracting the interest of immunologists all over the world. But leprosy bacilli obtained from patients with different types of the disease, and living in different parts of the world, all produce identical histopathological changes when transmitted to the foot pads of mice, and this strongly suggests that human leprosy is produced by one strain of bacillus, and that clinical patterns of the disease are determined by different host responses, i.e. by immunological factors in the host.[1]

IMMUNOLOGY

The study of immunology is the study of the ways in which the body produces a defensive reaction to the presence of alien (foreign) substances which enter the body. We can call these alien substances antigens or immunogens, and the defensive reaction can be called the immune response or, simply, immunity. There are two principal defence mechanisms: one is a humoral immune response and the other is a cell-mediated immune response, the former depending on a group of small lymphocytes called B lymphocytes (B cells) and the latter depending on a group of small lymphocytes called T lymphocytes (T cells).

B cells and T cells

B cells originate in bone marrow and travel directly into lymphoid tissues (the 'secondary' or 'peripheral' lymphoid organs, such as spleen, lymph nodes and Peyer's patches) where they constitute the major part of the small lymphocyte population; in the spleen they occupy the red pulp, in the lymph nodes they occupy the germinal centres (lymphoid follicles) and the medullary cords, and a relatively small proportion can be found in the bloodstream. T cells also originate in bone marrow, but unlike B cells they do not travel directly into lymphoid tissues but first enter the thymus (the 'primary' or 'central' lymphoid organ) where they undergo a conditioning process, hence the name thymus-dependent lymphocytes. After leaving the thymus they migrate to special regions of lymph nodes and spleen known as thymus-dependent areas, namely, the paracortical areas of lymph nodes and the periarteriolar regions of the splenic white pulp, and have a special tendency to circulate from one lymphoid organ to another in lymph and blood (the recirculating pool). 75–80% of blood lymphocytes are T cells, and 10–20% are B cells.[2] T and B cells cannot be differentiated among the small lymphocytes in a blood film routinely stained for a differential white cell count, but immunologists have devised methods of identification. For example, B cells have a surface immunoglobulin which can be visualised under the microscope by immunofluorescence.

THE HUMORAL IMMUNE RESPONSE

B cells within the lymphoid tissues of the body (spleen, lymph nodes, bone marrow, Peyer's patches and lamina propria of the gut) are stimulated by antigen to proliferate and transform into plasma cells, and the plasma cells, in turn, produce immunoglobulins. Immunoglobulins are serum proteins which possess antibody activity and which are classed according to the antigens which stimulate their production: immunoglobulin G (IgG), immunoglobulin M (IgM), immunoglobulin A (IgA), immunoglobulin D (IgD) and immunoglobulin E (IgE).

Four subclasses have been identified in IgG, namely, IgG1, IgG2, IgG3 and IgG4. In order for antibody to have a cytotoxic (cell-killing) effect, an extra protein substance is required; it is called complement, and much is now known about its nature and function.[3] Suffice it to say that complement is found in serum proteins and tissue fluids, and its activity in the humoral immune response results from the combined activity of nine complement component proteins numbered 1 to 9 (C1 to C9). However, there are eleven in all because C1 has three subcomponents: C1q, C1r and C1s. As has been said, B cells are essential in the humoral immune response, but a word must be said about the part played by T cells in assisting or collaborating with B cells in the humoral mechanism. A subset of T cells known as helper or inducer T cells (T4 cells) are able, on activation by antigen, to release a 'helper' factor which enables B cells to respond to antigens which they otherwise would not recognise. Conversely, suppressor T cells (T8 cells) may in certain circumstances exert a regulating or 'suppressor' effect on B cells. These 'helper' and 'suppressor' factors are among a number of non-antibody proteins generated by lymphocyte activation and are known as lymphokines;[4] these play an important role in amplifying and modulating the lymphocyte–lymphocyte and lymphocyte–macrophage interactions by which humoral and cell-mediated responses are regulated, but 'it is not known whether the helper T cells that are required to initiate cell-mediated responses are identical to those that induce antibody synthesis in B cells'.[5]

THE HUMORAL IMMUNE RESPONSE IN LEPROSY

Humoral immune responses in leprosy appear to be unimpaired, for not only do patients usually have raised levels of serum immunoglobulins, but they are fully capable of forming antibodies to bacterial vaccines such as typhoid vaccine. Numerous workers have reported raised levels of IgG, IgM and IgA in all types of leprosy, with highest levels in LL, especially of IgG, and there are some reports of slightly raised IgE levels. Peripheral blood B cells, the producers of antibodies, are increased in LL. Specific antibodies against *M. leprae* have been demonstrated in LL, and these have been found in the IgG and IgM classes.[6] Unfortunately for the leprosy patient, the cell wall of *M. leprae* protects it against these specific circulating humoral antibodies; worse still, the antibodies may actually be harmful as they can react with *M. leprae* antigens in the tissues during the Type 2 lepra reaction (ENL reaction), with the deposition of immunoglobulin and complement (immune complexes) in the damaged tissues (see p. 89). Although there is little difference between the raised serum levels of immunoglobulin in LL in reaction and without reaction, complement (C2 and C3) is raised in the former. Immunologists now have several specific serological antibody tests giving positive results in most leprosy patients,[7] and as seropositivity precedes clinical diagnosis in all types of leprosy, particularly in LL patients who have very high antibody levels at time of diagnosis, use can be made of this in the identification of individuals progressing towards the lepromatous form of disease.[7] Furthermore, specific antibody tests have a place in diagnosing subclinical leprosy infection in exposed individuals in endemic areas. On this subject, Abe *et al.*,[8] in Japan, have introduced a fluorescent leprosy antibody absorption (FLA–ABS) test for detecting subclinical leprosy infection. They found 92% 'positives' in household contacts, mean antibody titres being highest in infants less than 4 years old and tending to decrease with increasing age – a possible indication that leprosy infection is most frequent in infancy. The test, by itself, does not indicate which of the 'positives' will develop clinical leprosy, but, taken in conjunction with the lepromin test, these workers suggest that those who have a positive lepromin test are not in danger whereas those with a negative lepromin test are at risk of developing overt leprosy. The test has proved highly sensitive in other lands.[9]

THE CELL-MEDIATED IMMUNE RESPONSE

T cells are essential in cell-mediated immunity (CMI) and can penetrate most tissues to mediate cellular immune reactions to antigen, and such reactions are important in transplant rejection, defence against malignant cells, and resistance to various infections. T cells responding to antigens undergo blast transformation (enlargement and division) and proliferate in the thymus-dependent regions of lymphoid tissue, particularly the paracortical areas of lymph nodes. Such activated T cells have a complex reaction with macrophages (phagocytic cells), one of which involves the release from T cells of soluble factors called lymphokines, such as migration-inhibiting factor (MIF) which immobilises or concentrates macrophages at sites where their activity is required, and macrophage-activating factor (MAF) which renders macrophages capable of killing micro-organisms or other types of invading cells, such as malignant cells.

Two *in vitro* methods of measuring T cell activity are the lymphocyte transformation test (LTT) and the leucocyte migration inhibition test (LMIT). In the LTT, T cells are stimulated to enlarge and divide, a phenomenon known as blast or blastoid transformation, after contact with mitogens, such as phytohaemagglutinin (PHA test), allogeneic lymphocytes (MLC test), or tuberculin (PPD), candida, mumps, etc. The LMIT is basically a test of the capacity of T cells to produce MIF on antigenic stimulation.

An *in vivo* method of testing for CMI is by injecting antigen intradermally and studying the local reaction after 48–72 hours. A vaccine can be used containing an antigen to which the patient has already been exposed, such as *Candida* extract or tuberculin (PPD), or chemicals, such as dinitrochlorobenzene (DNCB) or trinitrochlorobenzene ('picryl chloride') can also be used. This reaction, known as delayed hypersensitivity or delayed-type hypersensitivity (DH or DTH), is one which is closely interconnected with CMI. Graft versus host (GVH) reactions are a further means of assessing CMI, and details of such a reaction in leprosy are given below.

THE CELL-MEDIATED IMMUNE RESPONSE IN LEPROSY

Non-specific CMI in leprosy

This can be shown by delayed hypersensitivity (DH) reactions to various skin test antigens, and by the PHA-induced lymphocyte transformation test (LTT) which gives a negative or poor response in untreated LL and a normal response in TT. It is interesting that this test gives a normal response in long-treated and inactive LL. Another example of non-specific impaired CMI in leprosy is the delay in rejecting an allograft (a graft from another human); in TT, skin allografts survive for 2 days longer than in healthy persons, and in LL they survive 4 days longer on average. It should be noted, however, that non-specific impairment of CMI in leprosy is not associated with any predisposition to infection, whether viral, bacterial, protozoal or mycotic. As regards cancer, apart from a rare incidence of squamous cell carcinoma complicating chronic leg or plantar ulcer, it can be said that the leprosy patient has no predisposition to malignant disease. This has been shown in studies of cancer morbidity in leprosy patients in the USA[10,11] and in Japan.[12]

Specific CMI in leprosy

It is the deficient CMI and DH to *M. leprae* that are responsible for an individual developing leprosy as a result of contact with the bacterium, and it is the degree of deficiency which determines the type of leprosy (see Fig. 2.4, p. 22).

In vitro *tests of specific CMI*

Tests of delayed hypersensitivity (DH) to *M. leprae* One test is the *lymphocyte transformation test* (LTT) using *M. leprae* antigen. The test is negative in LL, strongly positive in TT, and gives an intermediate result in borderline leprosy. The negative response in untreated LL is not altered after prolonged treatment (compare with the non-specific test, p. 72). But increased responses have been obtained during upgrading (reversal) reactions in borderline leprosy, falling to the original levels, or lower, when reactions have subsided, even though clinical and histological improvement have been maintained.[13] It is generally agreed that the LTT, although useful in working with groups of patients, is not a reliable tool for evaluating individual patients.[14] The test shows no essential difference between LLp and LLs.[15] Using this test, Godal and Negassi[16] have shown a difference between healthy persons never exposed to leprosy and those who have for a long time been in contact with patients, the former group giving a negative or poor response and the latter group giving a good response. But these workers found a relatively low response in those in close domestic contact with active lepromatous patients, i.e. during the first 6 months of treatment; they suggested that 'in these contacts "superexposure" to *M. leprae* can bring about a decrease in host resistance'.

The *lymphocyte stimulation test* (LST) is another test of lymphocyte stimulation, but instead of measuring the blastoid reaction in lymphocytes it records the radioactivity in the DNA fraction of lymphocytes after incorporation of labelled thymidine. It is more modern than the LTT and is generally considered less difficult to carry out. Various preparations of *M. leprae* have been used as antigen in these tests, including whole bacilli, heat-killed bacilli and various antigenic fractions of the organism. Applying the LST, and using a special antigen fraction prepared from *M. leprae*, Closs *et al.*[17] have shown that leprosy patients in the TT and BT groups had moderate or strong responses, and those in the BL and LL groups had weak or absent responses. Although there was a tendency towards stronger responses in the TT than in the BT group, the variation within each group was much more striking. Moreover, the highest responses in the BL group were higher than the lowest responses in the TT group, confirming that the LST, like the LTT, is unreliable in assessing the specific immunity of individual patients. However, they found that the distinction between healthy contacts of leprosy patients and non-exposed individuals was better than in a previous study using the LTT with whole *M. leprae* antigen.[18] Therefore it is a better test for subclinical infections, although it must be appreciated that it does not show which sublinical leprosy will become clinical and which will not.

Lymphokine production by T cells is a more reliable *in vitro* method of assessing CMI in leprosy, and records lymphokine production by T cells on cultivation with *M. leprae* and the effect on macrophages.[19] Macrophage activating factor (MAF) and migration inhibiting factor (MIF) have been produced in TT but not in LL, showing a lack of macrophage activation in LL and consequent failure to kill *M. leprae* within macrophages. Many healthy persons living in regions where leprosy is endemic can produce MIF when their lymphocytes are incubated with *M. leprae*, suggesting that subclinical infections are more common than clinically manifest disease; a conclusion which has already been reached from studies of lymphocyte stimulation (LTT and LST). Leprosy, therefore, is a disease of high infectivity but low pathogenicity.

γ-Interferon (gamma or immune interferon) is the major component of MAF and is important in controlling viral infections. Its function in leprosy has been well described by Kaplan and Cohn:[20]

> 'Interferon-γ (IFN-γ) appears to be the principal factor secreted by antigen-stimulated lymphocytes that activates macrophages . . . Deficient macrophage activation may be a characteristic of borderline and polar lepromatous leprosy . . . we have shown that monocytes from the blood of lepromatous leprosy patients respond normally to recombinant IFN-γ with enhanced secretion of H_2O_2 . . . These observations have led us to conclude that the immune deficit in lepromatous leprosy probably results from a lack of response to *M. leprae* by the patients' T cells. This would result in a reduced or absent release of lymphokines including IFN-γ leading to a local lack of macrophage activation and the absence of killing of intracellular *M. leprae*.'

Interleukin-2 (IL-2) is a soluble T cell growth factor which is produced by activation of one of several T cell subpopulations (subsets) specialised to deal with various immune effector functions. It is important in the humoral defence mechanism by promoting antibody production from B cells, and its importance in the cell-mediated response to challenge by *M. leprae* has been shown by Haregewoin *et al.*[19] who were able to activate lepromatous T cells by *M. leprae* antigen when cultivated in a medium containing IL–2.

Helper (T4) and suppressor (T8) cells The presence of T4 and T8 cells in dermal lesions of leprosy has been studied by Kaplan and Cohn[20] who have shown that the great majority of the T cells found in lepromatous skin lesions are of the T8 (suppressor) subset, while very few T4 (helper) cells are present. These increase in numbers as one progresses towards TT. These authors write:

> 'The exuberant growth of *M. leprae* within macrophages of lepromatous lesions stands in striking contrast to the paucibacillary macrophages of tuberculoid leprosy. The permissive nature of the macrophages of the lepromatous lesions together with the selective absence of helper T cells suggested a lack of local lymphokine production and inadequate macrophage activation.'

In vivo *tests of specific CMI in leprosy*

The lepromin test This delayed hypersensitivity test is negative in LL, BL, and BB, is weakly positive in BT, and is strongly positive in TT. It has been fully described in Chapter 3.

Examination of lymph nodes In LL there is depletion of lymphocytes in the paracortical areas of lymph nodes and their replacement by macrophages, while in TT the active CMI is shown by the proliferation of lymphocytes in these areas.[21,22] In upgrading (reversal) reactions in borderline leprosy, where there is a rapid shift of CMI towards the tuberculoid pole of the spectrum, corresponding changes in lymph nodes have been demonstrated.

Graft versus host reaction This method of assessing CMI has been demonstrated by Mehra and colleagues.[23] They injected peripheral blood lymphocytes intravenously into immunologically suppressed mice, and measured the rate of blastoid transformation of the donor cells by the radioactive thymidine uptake in the periarteriolar areas of the spleen; the number of cells labelled with thymidine was highest in healthy persons (paramedical personnel working among patients), slightly less in tuberculoid patients, still less in borderline patients, and least of all in those suffering from lepromatous leprosy. All were untreated at the time. However, a group with inactive (long-treated) LL, similarly tested, revealed an enhanced rate of blastoid transformation and thymidine uptake, suggesting that the suppression of CMI in LL may not be a permanent phenomenon, being only secondary to the excessive mycobacterial antigen load.

MONOCLONAL ANTIBODIES (MABs)

A short note on this subject is being included so that readers will not be puzzled when they come across the term in leprosy journals. To immunologists, the subject of monoclonal antibodies is of absorbing interest, and it has been discussed by Ivanyi.[24] He explains that until recently immunological investigations on humoral and cell-mediated reactions to *M. leprae* have concentrated on the response of the immune system *in toto*, with only scant attention to the fact that diverse reactions may arise towards the antigenic determinants (epitopes) of the various protein, glycolipid and polysaccharide constituents of *M. leprae*, and modern work with MABs will greatly contribute to the identification of those antigens which are functionally important for the development and progression of the respective forms of leprosy.

Whereas polyclonal antibodies from immunised individuals are derived from multiple clones of B cells, MABs are the product of a single B lymphocyte clone which has been 'immortalised' by fusion with an autonomously growing myeloma cell. They are uniform in specificity and structure, and each MAB can identify one antigenic determinant, and one only, within or on the surface of *M. leprae*. It is anticipated that, in addition to their already established functions,[25] MABs will be the method of choice in differentiating *M. leprae* from other acid-fast mycobacteria.

AETIOLOGICAL FACTORS IN LEPROSY

It is generally accepted that the outcome of infection with *M. leprae* depends on the integrity of the host's specific cellular immune response, but the reason or reasons for diminished CMI to *M. leprae*, resulting in overt disease, are not known. A variety of possible factors have been postulated by immunologists only to be contradicted by others. Among the possibilities which have been studied, without firm conclusions being drawn, are:

1 *Genetic constitution* – Studies on twins have not given unequivocal support to the view that there is a genetic factor in susceptibility to leprosy.[26] Recent researches have concentrated on a possible association between leprosy and HLA haplotype, and early work with HLA-A and HLA-B types suggested that siblings with the same type of leprosy had significant excess of identical HLA type, whereas siblings with different types of leprosy did not.[27] But a later study of HLA-D type in siblings[28] found that the development of LL was not under HLA-D control.

2 *A primary fault in T cells* – A primary fault could render them unable to stimulate macrophages, but *in vitro* tests have shown that LL patients possess functioning T cells.[19]

3 *A primary fault in macrophages* – This could render them unable to respond to T cell stimulation. However, among a number of findings against this hypothesis is the fact that the inability of lepromatous macrophages to respond *in vitro* to *M. leprae* antigen when on their own, or in the presence of lepromatous lymphocytes, can be reversed if lymphocytes from TT patients are present.[29] This was demonstrated in a modified macrophage migration-inhibition test, and proved that macrophages from LL patients could respond to MIF.

4 *Suppressor cell activity* – Recently, there has been much discussion on the existence of subpopulations of T cells which decrease immune responses (suppressor cells). However, in a review of this important hypothesis by Rook[30] it is concluded that there is inadequate support for the concept that inappropriate suppressor cell activity contributes to the pathogenesis of leprosy. It has been suggested by Turk[31] that the many contradictory observations may be due to different responses in patients from different ethnic groups.

5 *Abnormal antigen presentation* – The normal way for effective CMI to *M. leprae* to be induced is by leakage of bacillary antigens to the peripheral lymphon compartment (regional lymph nodes), via lymphatic vessels. But, if antigens are first presented to the central lymphon compartment (spleen, thymus, bone-marrow) via the bloodstream, a humoral immune response results and is accompanied by suppressed cellular response. Stoner[32] has described how the neural predilection of *M. leprae* results in a continuous leakage of leprosy bacilli

into the circulation; this is because there are no true lymphatics within the nerve fasciculus (funiculus), and as the perineurium is an effective barrier to epineurial lymphatic channels, leprosy bacilli are barred from the peripheral lymphon compartment.

IMMUNOPROPHYLAXIS AND IMMUNOTHERAPY IN LEPROSY

Immunoprophylaxis

A report on the efficacy of BCG vaccine in leprosy is given in Chapter 11, p. 147, and shows that it has limitations. However, until such time as a specific vaccine becomes available, the authors recommend that it be given to all children in endemic areas of leprosy, especially to newborn infants. As regards a specific vaccine, laboratory research and field trials are proceeding as part of the WHO Immunology of Leprosy (IMMLEP) programme, and the vaccines of greatest promise are: (a) a vaccine combining killed *M. leprae* with live BCG, based on the successful trials by Convit *et al.* in Venezuela.[33] (b) A vaccine containing the ICRG bacillus inactivated by γ-irradiation.[34] This bacterium which belongs to the *M. avium intracellulare* group of environmental acid-fast mycobacteria is one of many which have been cultivated from human lepromata,[35] and shows great cross reactivity with *M. leprae*. One vaccine containing this bacillus on its own, and one combined with BCG, are undergoing field trials in India.[34] One advantage of including BCG in the vaccine is its value in protection against tuberculosis.

Immunotherapy

A list of trials of various kinds was given in the previous edition of this book, but even the most promising – the giving of intravenous injections of transfer factor (TF) – has proved disappointing.[36] The method of real promise is that devised by Convit and colleagues in Venezuela.[37] They use a vaccine containing killed *M. leprae* and living BCG to generate CMI in patients with indeterminate leprosy who are Mitsuda-negative, and in BL and LL patients. They give the vaccine intradermally in three sites (both deltoid regions and the upper back), and this is repeated, if required, three or more times at intervals of 2–3 months. Chemotherapy need not be interrupted.

The use of levamisole, a chemical modulator to increase CMI, has yet to be established in leprosy. It can be anticipated that research into AIDS, and its associated depressed CMI, will provide new methods of improving CMI which can be applied in the immunotherapy of leprosy.

REFERENCES

1 Rees R. J. W. (1965). Recent bacteriologic, immunologic and pathologic studies on experimental human leprosy in the mouse foot pad. *International Journal of Leprosy*; **33**: 646–55.

2 Holborow E. J., Papamichael M. (1983). The lymphoid system and lymphocytic subpopulations. In *Immunology in Medicine* (Holborow E. J., Reeves W. G., eds.) pp. 17–34. London, New York: Grune and Stratton.

3 Thompson R. A. (1983). Complement. In *Immunology and Medicine* (Holborow E. J., Reeves W. G., eds) pp. 95–119. London, New York: Grune and Stratton.

4 Dumonde D. C., Hamblin A. (1983). Lymphokines. In *Immunology and Medicine* (Holborow E. J., Reeves W. G., eds) pp. 121–50. London, New York: Grune and Stratton.

5 Watson J. D., Booth R. J. (1987). The potential role of DNA technology in leprosy. *Leprosy Review*; **58**: 201–6.

6 World Health Organization (1973). Immunological problems in leprosy research: 1. Reprinted in *Leprosy Review* (1974); **45**: 244–56.

7 Editorial (1986). Serological tests for leprosy. *Lancet*; **i**: 533–5.

8 Abe M., Minagawa F., Yoshino Y., Ozawa T., Saikawa K., Saito T. (1980). Fluorescent leprosy antibody absorption (FLA–ABS) test for detecting subclinical infection with *Mycobacterium leprae*. *International Journal of Leprosy*; **48**: 109–19.

9 Bharadwaj V. P., Ramu G., Desikan K. V., Katoch K. (1984). Extended studies on subclinical infection in leprosy. *Indian Journal of Leprosy*; **56**: 807–12.

10 Oleinick A. (1969). Altered immunity and cancer risk: a review of the problem and analysis of the cancer mortality experience in leprosy patients. *Journal of the National Cancer Institute*; **43**: 775–81.
11 Brinton L. A., Hoover R., Jacobson R. R., Fraumeni J. F. Jnr. (1984). Cancer mortality among patients with Hansen's Disease. *Journal of the National Cancer Institute*; **72**: 109–14.
12 Tokudome S., Kono S., Ikeda M., Kuratsune M., Kumamaru S. (1981). Cancer and other causes of death among leprosy patients. *Journal of the National Cancer Institute*; **67**: 285–9.
13 Bjune G., Barnetson R. St C., Ridley D. S., Kronvall G. (1976). Lymphocyte transformation test in leprosy: correlation of the response with inflammation of lesions. *Clinical and Experimental Immunology*; **25**: 85–94.
14 Ridley D. S. (1976). Hypersensitivity and immunity reactions and classification. *Leprosy Review*; **47**: 171–4.
15 Myrvang B., Godal T., Ridley D. S., Fröland S. S., Song Y. K. (1973). Immune responsiveness to *Mycobacterium leprae* and other mycobacterial antigens throughout the clinical and histopathological spectrum of leprosy. *Clinical and Experimental Immunology*; **14**: 541–53.
16 Godal T., Negassi K. (1973). Subclinical infection in leprosy. *British Medical Journal*; **3**: 557–9.
17 Closs O., Reitan L. J., Negassi K., Harboe M., Belehu A. (1982). In vitro stimulation of lymphocytes in leprosy patients, healthy contacts of leprosy patients, and subjects not exposed to leprosy: comparison of an antigen fraction prepared from *Mycobacterium leprae* and tuberculin purified protein derivative. *Scandinavian Journal of Immunology*; **16**: 103–15.
18 Godal T., Loftgren M., Negassi K. (1972). Immune response to *M. leprae* of healthy contacts. *International Journal of Leprosy*; **40**: 243.
19 Haregewoin A., Godal T., Mustafa A. S., Belehu A., Yemaneberhan T. (1983). T-cell conditioned media reverse T-cell unresponsiveness in lepromatous leprosy. *Nature*; **303**: 342–4.
20 Kaplan G., Cohn Z. A. (1986). Regulation of cell-mediated

immunity in lepromatous leprosy. *Leprosy Review*; **57 (suppl. 2)**: 199–202.
21 Desikan K. V. (1974). Morphological changes in the lymph nodes in leprosy with special reference to the unstable forms. *Leprosy in India*; **46**: 35–8.
22 Waters M. F. R., Turk J. L., Wemambu S. N. C. (1971). Mechanisms of reactions in leprosy. *International Journal of Leprosy*; **39**: 417–28.
23 Mehra N. K., Dasgupta A., Vaidya M. C. (1976). An evaluation of the immune state in leprosy. *Leprosy in India*; **48**: 231–7.
24 Ivanyi J. (1984). Application of monoclonal antibodies towards immunological studies in leprosy. *Leprosy Review*; **55**: 1–9.
25 Sengupta U., Sinha S. (1984). Monoclonal antibodies against *Mycobacterium leprae* and their applications in leprosy research. *Indian Journal of Leprosy*; **56**: 727–41.
26 Chakravartti M. R., Vogel F. (1973). A twin study on leprosy. In *Topics in Human Genetics*, Vol.1. (Becker P. E. *et al.*, eds). Stuttgart: Georg Thième Verlag.
27 de Vries R. R. P., Nijenhuis L. E., van Rood J. J. (1976). HLA-linked genetic control of host response to *Mycobacterium leprae*. *Lancet*; **ii**: 1328–30.
28 Stoner G. L., Touw J., Belehu A., Naafs B. (1978). In-vitro lymphoproliferative response to *Mycobacterium leprae* of HLA-D-identical siblings of lepromatous leprosy patients. *Lancet*; **ii**: 543–7.
29 Han S. H., Weiser R. S., Wang J. J., Tsai L. C., Lin P. P. (1974). The behavior of leprous lymphocytes and macrophages in the macrophage migration-inhibition test. *International Journal of Leprosy*; **42**: 186–91.
30 Rook G. A. W. (1982). Suppressor cells of mouse and man. What is the evidence that they contribute to the aetiology of the mycobacterioses? *Leprosy Review*; **53**: 306–12.
31 Turk J. L. (1982). Immunopathology of Leprosy. In *Critical Reviews in Tropical Medicine*, Vol.1 (Chandra R. K., ed) pp. 143–69. New York, London: Plenum Press.
32 Stoner G. L. (1979). Importance of the neural predilection of *Mycobacterium leprae* in leprosy. *Lancet*; **ii**: 994–6.
33 Convit J., Aranzazu N., Ulrich M., Zuniga M., de Aragon

M. E., Alvarado J. (1983). Investigations related to the development of a leprosy vaccine. *International Journal of Leprosy*; **51**: 531–9.

34 Deo M. G. (1984). Anti-leprosy vaccines – field trials and future prospects. *Indian Journal of Leprosy*; **56**: 764–75.

35 Draper P. (1983). Leprosy Review: the bacteriology of *Mycobacterium leprae*. *International Journal of Leprosy*; **51**: 563–75.

36 Faber W. R., Leiker D. L., Nengerman I. M., Schellekens P.Th.A. (1978). A placebo controlled clinical trial of transfer factor in lepromatous leprosy. In *Leprosy – Proceedings of the XI International Leprosy Congress* (Latapi F. *et al.*, eds) pp. 324–5. Amsterdam: Excerpta Medica.

37 Convit. J., Aranzazu N., Ulrich M., Pinardi M. E., Reyes O., Alvardo J. (1982). Immunotherapy with a mixture of *Mycobacterium leprae* and BCG in different forms of leprosy and in Mitsuda-negative contacts. *International Journal of Leprosy*; **50**: 415–24.

6 Leprosy Reactions (Reactional States)

In 1959 one of the authors (WHJ)[1] made an attempt to clarify the vexed subject of reactional leprosy, and this early classification was expanded in the first edition of this book[2] proposing the names Type 1 and Type 2 for the two major types of reaction, and using the term 'lepra reaction' to cover both types. But although this scheme has earned a good deal of support, some leprologists prefer to use the term lepra reaction to describe Type 1 reaction, and ENL reaction to describe Type 2. In view of the fact that immunologists accept four types of hypersensitivity (allergic) reactions (Types I–IV), it is suggested that the terms Type 1 lepra reaction and Type 2 lepra reaction be used in full should there be any possibility of confusion.

TYPE 1 LEPRA REACTION

This is a delayed hypersensitivity reaction which is an example of Coombs and Gell Type IV hypersensitivity reaction. Antigen from breaking down leprosy bacilli reacts with T lymphocytes and this is associated with a rapid change in cell-mediated immunity (CMI). It is typically seen in borderline patients because of their immunological instability, and if the reaction is associated with a rapid increase in specific CMI, as it is in patients under treatment, we speak of upgrading or reversal reaction (RR). This is because the natural tendency for borderline leprosy to downgrade slowly towards the lepromatous pole, in the absence of treatment, is reversed. On the other hand, if the reaction is associated with a reduction in immunity we speak of downgrading reaction. In BT and BB patients, the most likely time for upgrading reaction to occur is during the first 6 months of treatment, but longer intervals have been recorded in BL.[3] Sometimes a patient may be in reaction when first seen at the clinic. Upgrading reaction may also occur in sub-polar LL (LLs) under treatment; these patients rapidly regain lost immunity and the new skin lesions have the features of BL. Borderline patients may upgrade to the tuberculoid type (TT) but form a subgroup – secondary tuberculoid or TTs[4] – which, in contrast to its counterpart at the other end of the spectrum (sub-polar LL or LLs) appears to be immunologically stable. Upgrading reactions are better documented than downgrading ones, and one reason is that patients under treatment are more likely to have their progress observed. The various shifts across the leprosy spectrum are: LLs → BL → BB → BT → TTs. LLp and TTp, the polar forms, are immunologically stable. The reverse holds good in downgrading reactions: BT → BB → BL → LLs.

Clinically, the most prominent sign is a rapidly-developing change in the appearance of some or all the skin lesions; they become erythematous, more prominent, shiny, warm to touch, and resembling erysipelas (Plate 17). Sometimes necrosis supervenes with breakdown and ulceration. Lesions desquamate as they subside. The authors have seen a crop of new lesions appear on the skin as part of an upgrading reaction in borderline leprosy, and at first suspected that the reaction was downgrading, especially as the new lesions appeared shiny. However, upgrading was confirmed by histology and by lepromin testing. Systemic disturbance, such as malaise and fever is unusual, but nerve involvement is common. This takes the form of rapid swelling of one or more nerves with pain and tenderness at the site of nerve swelling, usually where the nerve is most superficial. Sometimes pain is referred to the region of the skin which a sensory nerve or a mixed nerve supplies, such as pain at the medial border of the wrist and/or in the little finger in ulnar nerve involvement; in such a case the ulnar nerve will be tender on palpation just above the elbow. More serious is motor disturbance, and the nerves most at risk are the ulnar (causing claw hand), the lateral popliteal (causing dropped foot), and the facial (causing facial palsy). Facial palsy is most likely to occur if there is a lesion on one cheek. These paralyses are likely to be permanent if neglected or incorrectly treated, but will recover with correct and prompt treatment. The cause of nerve pain is increased intraneural pressure from oedema and cellular reaction (granuloma formation), aggravated at sites where swollen nerve trunks are entrapped in bony or fascial tunnels, e.g. cubital tunnel and carpal tunnel syndromes. Rarely, a nerve abscess may form, producing a fluctuant swelling attached to the affected nerve. It is usually the ulnar nerve which is affected in this way, but the great auricular or the common peroneal (lateral popliteal) have also been known to be the only ones involved. Another associated manifestation is oedema of hands, feet, or face; sometimes all three sites are involved, or, rarely, one foot or one hand. Tenderness of palms and soles is often present, and may sometimes herald an upgrading reaction. Fever and malaise have been reported, but are unusual (compare Type 2 reaction).

The histological changes in Type 1 reaction are listed in Table 6.1, but for a full description of the histological course of reactions in borderline leprosy the paper by Ridley and Radia should be studied.[5] Immunological changes include alterations in lepromin reaction and in the reactivity of the lymphocyte transformation test (LTT) and lymphocyte stimulation test (LST) using *M. leprae* as antigen, and cellular changes in the paracortical regions of lymph nodes (see Chapter 5).

TYPE 2 LEPRA REACTION

This type of reaction differs from reversal (upgrading) reaction in several ways. First, it is not associated with alteration in CMI as it is an immune complex syndrome (an antigen–antibody reaction involving complement) and thus is a humoral antibody response. It is an example of Type III hypersensitivity reaction (Coombs and Gell). Second, it occurs almost exclusively in lepromatous leprosy (LLp and LLs), only occasionally appearing in BL. Third, the clinician sees no change whatsoever in the appearance of the leprosy lesions (even though the histologist may see some evidence of change), but may see crops of brightly erythematous nodules which come and go. These are not observed in upgrading reaction. Fourth, systemic disturbance is usual (the patient may be pyrexial and toxic – see Fig. 9.1, p. 123). Fifth, unlike upgrading reaction, when it occurs in relation to therapy (as it often does), it is very unusual for it to occur during the first 6 months of therapy. It tends to occur later during the course of treatment when skin lesions appear quiescent and all or most of the bacilli in the skin are granular. However, a patient may be in reaction when first seen,

Table 6.1 Classification of lepra reaction (reaction in leprosy)

Name of reaction	*Types of leprosy involved*	*Main clinical features*	*Main histological features (in dermis)*	*Main haematological findings*
Type 1 reaction	1 Borderline 2 Sub-polar lepromatous (LLs)	Erythema and swelling of some or all the leprosy skin lesions. New lesions may appear. Oedema of extremities. Neuritis.*	In reversal reaction there is oedema, reduced bacilli, and increased defensive cells, such as lymphocytes, epithelioid cells and giant cells. In downgrading reaction there is increase in bacilli, and defensive cells are replaced by macrophages.	Nil
Type 2 reaction	1 Lepromatous (LLp and LLs) 2 Some cases of BL (BL/LL)	Any of the following, singly or in various combinations: ENL, neuritis,* bone pain, joint pain, dactylitis, fever, malaise, lymphadenitis, rhinitis, epistaxis, iritis, epididymo-orchitis, proteinuria. In severe cases, ENL lesions may become vesicular or bullous and break down (erythema necroticans).	In ENL lesions there is oedema, neutrophil infiltration and sometimes vasculitis (veins and arterioles). In erythema necroticans there is obliterative angiitis and endarteritis. Bacilli are fragmented and granular.	Polymorphonuclear leucocytosis. Raised ESR. Thrombocytosis. Raised IgG, IgM, C2 and C3. Normocytic normochromic anaemia.

* Neuritis means nerve pain and swelling; anaesthesia and/or muscle paralysis may be associated.

either Type 1 or 2. Most leprologists would consider this unusual, but there has been a publication from Los Angeles reporting a series of 32 adults presenting for the first time, and 22 (69%) presented with ENL.[6] The term ENL reaction has been in use for a long time because of the crops of *erythema nodosum leprosum* (ENL) which often are present. However, because of the numerous symptoms in addition to ENL, some of which may occur in the absence of ENL, the authors prefer the name 'Type 2 reaction'. In other words, the new name covers all the manifestations of the symptom-complex rather than a particular one, and the name ENL can be reserved for the erythema nodosum lesions when they occur. It should be remembered that the first clinical and histological description of these lesions was given by a Japanese leprologist, Murata, in a German journal of pathology in 1912,[7] and when he proposed the name *erythema nodosum leprosum* it was for these lesions, not for the symptom-complex.

Erythema nodosum leprosum lesions are brightly erythematous, slightly raised nodules or plaques, variable in size but usually small, and if multiple tend to be distributed bilaterally and symmetrically (Plate 19). They are often tender, warmer than the surrounding skin, and blanch with light finger pressure (the red colour reappearing immediately pressure is released). They differ clinically from the type of erythema nodosum seen in conditions such as tuberculosis, sarcoidosis and acute rheumatism, by the fact that they are evanescent (lasting only 2 or 3 days, rarely longer), they can be very numerous, and can appear on regions of skin other than the lower legs. For example, they commonly occur on the face, arms and thighs; the flexor aspects of forearms and the medial aspects of thighs are favoured. In fact, they may appear on any skin area except the hairy scalp, axillae, groins and perineum; these are the warmer regions of skin which are avoided by leprosy lesions as well as by ENL. The authors have occasionally seen them on palms and soles. When they fade they leave a blue stain in the skin. When ENL lesions are numerous there is likely to be fever and malaise, the fever being intermittent with its fastigium in the evenings (Fig. 9.1, p. 123), and it is usual to find fresh crops of ENL lesions appearing between 17.00 and 18.00 hours, a time when endogenous cortisol production is at its lowest. They desquamate as they subside. The old-standing leprosy lesions, which were present when the reaction began, do not undergo any clinical change, and it is unusual for ENL lesions to be superimposed on them. In severe Type 2 reaction, ENL lesions may become vesicular or bullous and break down (erythema necroticans) (Plate 18). Often there is oedema of face, hands and feet. The classic histological features of active ENL lesions are, in the upper dermis, increased vascularity with many dilatated capillaries, and in the lower dermis intense infiltration with polymorphonuclear leucocytes (neutrophils) which have a predilection for surrounding blood vessels and invading their walls. There is swelling and oedema of the lining (endothelium) of veins, arterioles and small arteries in the ENL lesions. Swelling of endothelium, together with neutrophil infiltration of vessel walls is known as vasculitis. In erythema necroticans the invaded blood vessels undergo necrosis and obliteration of lumen (obliterative angiitis and endarteritis). Bacilli in ENL lesions are not as numerous as in the patient's leprosy lesions, and are mostly fragmented and granular. Any or all of the following symptoms and signs may be associated with ENL, or may occur without ENL, and all are manifestations of Type 2 reaction: fever and malaise, nerve pain, periosteal pain (especially in tibiae), muscle pain (myositis), pain and swelling in joints,[8] rhinitis, epistaxis, acute iritis (iridocyclitis), painful dactylitis, swollen and tender lymph nodes (especially femorals), acute epididymo-orchitis, and proteinuria. One of the authors (WHJ) has heard pericardial friction on auscultating the heart. A painful nerve trunk will be swollen and tender on palpation. Bone pain is usually confined to the tibiae, and there is exquisite tenderness (and a boggy feel) when palpated. Iritis may be unilateral or bilateral and can be mistaken for conjunctivitis, especially as it may occur on its own (without any other signs of reaction). As the treatment of these two conditions is radically different, and as delay in treating acute iritis can have serious consequences for the patient, it is important for leprosy workers to know how to differentiate them. In iritis the redness is most marked at the corneoscleral margin, i.e. where the central coloured part of the eye, covered by transparent cornea, joins the sclera (the white part of the eye). Further out the redness is paler or may be absent. Also, the redness is less intense than in conjunctivitis and tends to have a dusky or even a violet hue. The redness in conjunctivitis is most evident further out, and a useful aid to remembering this is to think of the letter 'i' for inland and the letter 'c' for coast; in iritis the

Table 6.2 Clinical aspects of conjunctivitis and iridocyclitis

Symptoms and signs	*Conjunctivitis*	*Iridocyclitis*
History of trauma or irritation	Common	No
Blurring of vision	No	Yes
Photophobia	No	Yes
Type of pain	No real pain. There may be an itchy or gritty sensation	Deep pain in the affected eye or eyes
Tint of redness	Bright red	Redness is less intense and has a dusky or maybe violet hue
Distribution of redness	More peripheral	More central
Exudate (discharge)	Usually present	Nil
Tender on palpatation	No	Yes
Pupil size and response	Normal	Small. Reactions are sluggish or absent

Modified from *Care of the Eye in Hansen's Disease* by Margaret Brand (revised 2nd ed. 1987). Obtainable free of charge from: Training Branch, Gillis W. Long Hansen's Disease Center, Carville, Louisiana 70721, USA.

redness is mostly 'inland' and in conjunctivitis it is mostly 'coastal'. See Table 6.2 for a comparison of the clinical aspects of conjunctivitis and iridocyclitis. Epididymo-orchitis may be unilateral or bilateral, the testis being swollen and acutely tender. Protein and red blood cells in the urine are likely to be manifestations of acute glomerulonephritis, for immune complexes have been demonstrated in renal glomeruli during Type 2 reaction,[9] and other workers have seen subepithelial humps, typical of immune glomerulonephritis, on electron microscopy.[10] Immune complexes have also been found by fluorescence microscopy in ENL lesions[11,12] thus likening ENL to the Arthus phenomenon, a condition which is known to be due to the deposition of immune complexes in and around the blood vessel walls. Wemambu *et al.*[12] found immunoglobulin and complement only in early ENL lesions, and they point out that such deposits may not be found in Arthus reactions examined 24 hours after their induction in laboratory animals. Some of the manifestations of Type 2 reaction have been likened to chronic serum sickness which is known to be associated with the presence of immune complexes in the circulation, for circulating immune complexes have been described during Type 2 reaction.[13,14] Other evidence of humoral antibody production can be found in positive tests for autoantibodies, such as rheumatoid factor and antinuclear factor. There is also an increase in circulating gammaglobulin with raised levels of IgG, IgM, C2 and C3.

The essential features of the two types of lepra reaction are shown in Table 6.1. The immunopathology of ENL has been described by Ridley and Ridley.[15]

Factors known to precipitate Type 2 reaction are: intercurrent infection, injury, surgical operation, physical stress, mental stress, protective immunisations (especially successful vaccination against smallpox), a strongly positive Mantoux test, pregnancy and parturition, ingestion of potassium iodide and of antileprosy drugs.

LUCIO'S PHENOMENON

This is a type of reaction confined to the diffuse non-nodular form of LL which is chiefly encountered in Mexicans, and among its unique features is the fact that it is seen only in untreated patients. This diffuse form of leprosy and its peculiar reaction were first described by Lucio and Alvarado in Mexico in 1852; they called this reaction 'lepra manchada'. In 1948, Latapi and Zamora[16] brought the original paper to the notice of the medical world, and they added their own observations: painful and tender red patches appear on the skin, particularly on the extremities, they become purpuric (the colour not disappearing on pressure), the centre of the purpuric lesion becomes necrotic and ulcerated and finally develops a brown or black crust (eschar) which falls off after a few days to leave a superficial atrophic scar. On the legs, the ulceration is larger and more lasting, with jagged edges surrounded by an inflammatory zone. Rea and Levan[17] have described the clinical, laboratory and histological findings in ten Mexican patients seen in the USA. They found the reacting lesions to be most common on the legs and less commonly on thighs, forearms and buttocks; trunk and face were spared. The patients were all untreated when their reactions developed, and were afebrile throughout. Although steroids had a good effect, thalidomide was of no value; good results were obtained with dapsone, and excellent results

1940s, and, until recent years, in low dosage. The first report was in 1964,[3] and since then there has been a steady increase in dapsone resistance worldwide, creating a serious problem which has been reviewed by Pearson.[4] The type of resistance which develops as a result of long-term monotherapy is secondary resistance, and is largely confined to LL because of the absence of CMI and the very long treatment. Drug-resistant mutants in the bacterial population develop in a stepwise manner with a multistep type mutation occurring in dapsone resistance (as in penicillin resistance), whereas a single-step mutation occurs in rifampicin resistance (as in streptomycin resistance). Resistant bacilli usually constitute only a part of the bacterial population, and in the case of dapsone are likely to be 'high resistant' mutants in patients who have relapsed while taking optimal dosage, and 'low-resistant' mutants for those who were on low dosage. 'Low-resistant' strains will be killed by optimal dosage of dapsone, but if such doses (100 mg/day) are given as monotherapy, fully resistant strains will develop in due course.

Primary resistance occurs in persons who are infected by dapsone-resistant *M. leprae*, and the first case, diagnosed clinically, occurred in Colombia.[5] The following year (1978) a proven case was reported from Malaysia[6] and another from India.[7] In contrast to secondary resistance, primary resistance may occur in any type of leprosy. Turning to more-recently introduced antileprosy drugs, the first report of rifampicin resistance was in 1976,[8] and the first report of clofazimine resistance was in 1982.[9]

Mouse foot pad inoculation is the method of proving drug resistance, and this involves counting the number of bacilli injected. Inocula must not contain more than 10^4 organisms (10 000), for multiplication fails when 10^5 or more are inoculated.[10] Inoculated mice are fed various concentrations of the drug to be tested. In the absence of drug resistance, bacilli multiply to a total of 10^6 by 6 months, after which no further multiplication takes place. If there is drug resistance multiplication is either modified or absent, depending on the daily dose incorporated in the food. There is increasing evidence that the level of resistance revealed by such techniques (referred to as partial or low, intermediate or full) is of considerable significance with regard to the likelihood of success or failure of continued full-dose dapsone therapy.[11]

Bacterial persistence

This is a phenomenon which can be defined as the capability of microorganisms to survive in the host irrespective of adequate antimicrobial treatment. It has been observed during infection with various bacteria, including *M. leprae* and *M. tuberculosis*. Persisting organisms were given the name 'persisters' by Bigger[12] when he was investigating the response of staphylococcal infections to penicillin. In leprosy the problem is peculiar to the treatment of LL, and small numbers of viable dapsone-sensitive 'persisters' have been isolated from patients treated with dapsone for 10–12 years,[13] and in patients treated with rifampicin for 2–5 years.[14] Sites favoured by 'persisters' are peripheral nerves, smooth muscle (e.g. dartos), and striated muscle (e.g. triceps). This important subject has been reviewed by Toman[15] who comes to the depressing conclusion that 'there is little reason to believe that, in the near future, a new drug or combination of drugs will be found that is capable of eradicating persisting *M. leprae*.'

REFERENCES

1 Brandsma J. W., de Jong N., Tjepkema T. (1986). Disability grading in leprosy. Suggested modifications to the WHO disability grading form. *Leprosy Review*; **57**: 361–9.

2 Karat A. B. A., Job C. K., Karat S., Rao G. S., Rao P. S. S. (1967). Domiciliary treatment programme absentee survey. *Leprosy in India*; **39**: 180–9.

3 Pettit J. H. S., Rees R. J. W. (1964). Sulphone resistance in leprosy: an experimental and clinical study. *Lancet*; **ii**: 673–4.

4 Pearson J. M. H. (1981). The problem of dapsone-resistant leprosy. *International Journal of Leprosy*; **49**: 417–20.

5 Londoño F. (1977). Primary sulphone resistance. *Leprosy Review*; **48**: 51.

6 Waters M. F. R., Laing A. B. G., Rees R. J. W. (1978). Proven primary dapsone resistance in leprosy – a case report. *Leprosy Review*; **49**: 127–30.

7 Girdhar B. K., Sreevatsa, Desikan K. V. (1978). Primary sulphone resistance. *Leprosy in India*; **50**: 352–5.

8 Jacobson R. R., Hastings R. C. (1976). Rifampin-resistant leprosy. *Lancet*; **ii**: 1304–5.

9 Warndorff-van Diepen T. (1982). Clofazimine-resistant lep-

rosy, a case report. *International Journal of Leprosy*; **50**: 139–42.

10 THELEP controlled clinical trials in lepromatous leprosy. (1983). *Leprosy Review*; **54**: 167–76.

11 *Laboratory Techniques for Leprosy* (1986). WHO/CDS/LEP/86.4. Geneva: WHO.

12 Bigger J. W. (1944). Treatment of staphylococcal infections with penicillin. *Lancet*; **ii**: 497–500.

13 Waters M. F. R., Rees R. J. W., McDougall A. C., Weddell A. G. M. (1974). Ten years of dapsone in lepromatous leprosy: clinical, bacteriological and histological assessment and the findings of viable leprosy bacilli. *Leprosy Review*; **45**: 288–98.

14 Rees R. J. W., Waters M. F. E., Pearson J. M. H., Helmy H. S., Laing A. B. G. (1976). Long-term treatment of dapsone-resistant leprosy with rifampicin: clinical and bacteriological studies. *International Journal of Leprosy*; **44**: 159–69.

15 Toman K. (1981). Bacterial persistence in leprosy. *International Journal of Leprosy*; **49**: 205–17.

8 Chemotherapy

Prior to initiating chemotherapy, and in addition to recording the patient's skin lesions and nerve involvement, a general examination should be carried out, including an eye examination, so that any associated disease can be treated. Investigations should include a urine and stool examination, blood count and chest x-ray. The following drugs, suitable in various combinations in the treatment of leprosy, will be described: dapsone, clofazimine, rifampicin, ethionamide and thiacetazone.

Table 8.1 Shelf-life of four antileprosy drugs

Drug	*Shelf-life*
Dapsone	4 years
Clofazimine	5 years
Rifampicin	4 years
Ethionamide/prothionamide	5 years

STORAGE OF TABLETS AND CAPSULES IN THE TROPICS

Tablets and capsules should be kept in firmly closed containers and shielded from light; if in glass containers, the glass should be dark. They should be kept as cool as possible, but not refrigerated. Capsules are a special problem as in hot and humid climates they tend to become gummed together. If storage in a silica gel bag is not possible, a simple method has been described by Dr Jon Wok Lee (1986) in *Leprosy Review*; **57**: 182. His method is to crush a tablet of dapsone into a fine powder and on shaking the powder with the capsules it acts as a separating 'talc' in the container.

DAPSONE (DDS; 4:4[1] DIAMINODIPHENYL SULPHONE)

The first effective treatment for leprosy was a sulphone named Promin (glucosulphone sodium), and this pioneer work was reported from Carville, USA, in 1943.[1] It had the disadvantage of having to be administered intravenously. Dapsone was introduced later in the 1940s by Cochrane and Muir in India, Lowe and Davey in Nigeria, and Souza Lima in Brazil.

The history of dapsone prior to the development of bacterial resistance is a brilliant success story covering a period exceeding 20 years. When we realise that the ingestion of one tablet of 100 mg gives, after about 4 hours, a peak blood level that is 500–600 times the minimum inhibitory concentration (MIC), and measurable amounts can be found in the blood 10 days later, we need not be surprised that it had such a long unbroken reign. Dapsone acts by inhibiting folate metabolism in *M. leprae*.[2] Dosage is 6–10 mg/kg of body weight per week, adults over 50 kg receiving 100 mg/day, while those under 50 kg receive 50 mg/day. Rarely it may be necessary to give dapsone by injection, and the pharmacy at University College Hospital, London, has overcome the problem of dapsone insolubility in water by dissolving it in alcohol and propylene glycol, a formula described by French.[3]

Dapsone	5 g
Absolute alcohol	40 ml
Benzyl alcohol	5 ml
Propylene glycol to	100 ml

This produces a solution of dapsone containing 50 mg in 1 ml, and intramuscular injections are painless. A preparation for intramuscular use is acedapsone, an acetyl derivative of dapsone made by Parke, Davis and Co. Other names are DADDS and Hansolar. It is a repository sulphone and 225 mg (1·5 ml) slowly releases the equivalent of 2·4 mg of dapsone daily, and each injection is effective for 3 months. A case can be made for giving an injection at each three-monthly clinic attendance, provided that oral dapsone is a constituent of combined chemotherapy. This will not only ensure a therapeutic level of dapsone in those who are irregular on self-administration of tablets, but patients in developing countries hold injections in high esteem and therefore are more likely to be regular on clinic attendances.

Side-effects of dapsone

Full details and references can be found in two[4,5] papers in *Leprosy Review.*

Effects on blood

Haemolysis of red blood cells is the most important of the side-effects of dapsone and should be suspected in any patient developing anaemia while on treatment. A study of the haemolytic effect of dapsone in normal men, and in men with deficiency of glucose-6-phosphate dehydrogenase (G-6-PD), confirmed that the latter were more susceptible to haemolysis, and there was a direct relationship between dosage and the extent of haemolysis in both groups.[6] Dapsone was found to be more haemolytic than primaquine in the normal group, and less so in the G-6-PD deficient group.

An additional factor in causing haemolysis is a toxic derivative of dapsone.[7] Dapsone is unrelated to iron-deficiency anaemia, so the only justification for giving iron with dapsone is that the iron will be useful in countering iron deficiency from other causes. Iron is not indicated in the treatment of haemolytic anaemia as it is liberated by the haemolysed red cells and retained in the body and stored for future use. Haemolysis is usually mild and symptomless on therapeutic dosage. Methaemoglobinaemia causes blueness of lips and fingernails, and will disappear spontaneously or on reduced dosage; on its own it is not an indication to interrupt therapy. A few cases of agranulocytosis have been recorded by dermatologists treating diseases other than leprosy, such as dermatitis herpetiformis which usually requires dosage in the region of 200–300 mg/day. However, the first report of agranulocytosis in treating leprosy appeared as recently as 1986[8] and the circumstances were tragic, not only because the patient died, but because he was being treated for indeterminate leprosy (see p. 45). A number of fatal cases of agranulocytosis occurred in US servicemen in Vietnam taking dapsone as a malaria prophylactic,[9] but dapsone's role is questionable as other antimalarials were being taken at the same time.[10] Thrombocytopenia is usually not severe enough to cause symptoms.

Effects on skin

A sensitivity reaction to dapsone is rare and takes the form of a symmetrical maculopapular rash sparing the face (exanthematous skin reaction), and it is fortunate that hypersensitivity skin reactions are rarer still, for they include exfoliative dermatitis, toxic epidermal necrolysis, Stevens–Johnson syndrome, and 'DDS' syndrome ('sulphone syndrome'). The last-named is likely to prove fatal and was described in the early years of dapsone's use when dangerously large doses were sometimes used; it disappeared during the decades when low dosage was in vogue, only to reappear in recent years. Fixed drug eruption may complicate treatment with dapsone after the drug has been well-tolerated by the patient for months or even years; it begins with one or more raised, erythematous, sharply demarcated, round or oval plaques which heal and become brown or black. The pathogenesis is obscure.[11]

Other side-effects

Peripheral neuropathy usually takes the form of a motor neuropathy with bilateral weakness of limbs, and tendon reflexes may be weak or absent. This side-effect has been recorded by dermatologists using doses larger than those used in leprosy. Psychosis is not uncommon in leprosaria where it has an incidence of about 10%, and as many factors are responsible it is very difficult to assess the role of dapsone, but rare cases have been reported in outpatients who have recovered on stopping the drug. Symptoms have included insomnia, irritability, delusions, and disordered thought and speech. A small minority of patients taking 100 mg/day complain that, an hour or two after taking the tablet, they feel temporarily 'woolly-headed' and unable to think clearly. This symptom improves if dosage is reduced, but before doing so it is worthwhile to try the effect of taking the 100 mg tablet on going to bed at night.

ENL and other manifestations of Type 2 reaction may be precipitated by dapsone (as by other antileprosy drugs), but these are not toxic effects as they are due to the killing of *M. leprae* and the release of antigen.

Should a pregnant woman take dapsone? The answer to this question is that no doctor likes giving drugs in the first trimester, but having regard to the importance of treating the patient's leprosy, and to the fact that countless numbers of pregnant women have taken dapsone without trouble, any theoretical risk can be ignored. Table 8.2 (p. 113) describes the possible ill effects of pregnancy, particularly if the leprosy is untreated.

Another advantage of treating the pregnant woman is that, in untreated LL, viable leprosy bacilli are present in breast milk. Thus, treatment during pregnancy will ensure that any bacilli in breast milk will be granular (dead). Clinicians working in developing countries are acquainted with a folic acid deficiency syndrome known as megaloblastic anaemia of pregnancy, and in view of dapsone's capacity to interfere with normal folate metabolism it would be wise to add folic acid 5 mg daily to patients receiving dapsone during pregnancy.

Serious effects of accidental overdose of dapsone have been reported, especially in children, and the importance of treatment with activated charcoal has been stressed.[12]

Testing for dapsone in the urine

A number of tests to monitor patient compliance have been described in recent years, and the one the authors can recommend for field use is the Spot test[13,14,15] developed by the late H. Huikeshoven on the early researches of de Castro in Brazil. The test involves placing a drop of fresh urine on a strip of filter paper impregnated with Ehrlich's reagent. A yellow ring appears at the periphery, caused by urea, and an inner spot of orange colour quickly develops when dapsone is present. The test is positive if the intensity of the central spot is equal to, or greater than, that given by the control urine.

(A booklet describing the spot test is available from Ingrid Kalf, Netherlands Leprosy Relief Association, Wibautstraat 135, 1097 DN Amsterdam, Netherlands.)

Manifestations of relapse in lepromatous leprosy

For a patient under treatment to present with *clinical* signs of relapse is a reproach for the medical team responsible for the patient's care, for had there been regular checks of progress by means of skin smears every 6 months, intimation of relapse would have been obtained long before clinical manifestations became obvious. Smears would have shown an increase in solid-staining bacilli, or the appearance of solid-staining bacilli when previously they had all been granular.

Clinical signs of relapse take the form of a few erythematous papulonodules which in the early stage are not likely to have the bilateral symmetrical distribution characteristic of well-established lepromatous leprosy, and tend to appear on unusual sites, such as the abdomen. It is important to avoid the mistake of thinking that they are ENL lesions by remembering that these disappear after a few days, while new ones appear at other sites. The way to test this is to mark one particular lesion and observe if it disappears; a leprosy nodule will appear unchanged. In addition, ENL lesions often are tender, and if pressed lightly by the examiner's finger their pink colour disappears only to return rapidly when the pressure is released. A smear from an ENL lesion contains relatively small numbers of granular bacilli, but many solid-staining bacilli are likely to be found in new and active leprosy nodules. A polymorphonuclear leucocytosis is indicative of ENL, as is an ESR over 50 mm in 1 hour, whereas in relapse there is no leucocytosis, the percentage of polymorphs is normal, and the ESR is below 50.

Post-treatment relapse in borderline leprosy has to be differentiated from Type 1 reaction, and this can be difficult. This is where experience in dealing with reaction is of the greatest value, for the experienced leprosy worker will suspect reaction if there is nerve pain and or tenderness, oedema of extremities, pyrexia, and if the new lesions are shiny, warm and desquamate as they subside.

CLOFAZIMINE (LAMPRENE; B663)

This red iminophenazine dye, first used by Browne and Hogerzeil[16] in the treatment of leprosy, is another drug that has proved its worth. In the 2nd edition of this book mention was made of its additional property of being effective as an anti-inflammatory agent in controlling the two types of lepra reaction; but this view must now be reconsidered. The present balance of opinion is that clofazimine is ineffective in Type 1 reaction, and unacceptably large doses are required over a long period of time to control ENL. Clofazimine's reputation for causing serious gastrointestinal side-effects has been gained almost entirely on this account. Therefore, it should be reserved for leprosy treatment in combination with other drugs. It is put up in capsules of 50 mg and 100 mg, and dosage is 300–350 mg/week, preferably administered as a daily capsule of 50 mg.

Side-effects

These are: red–brown pigmentation of skin and conjunctivae, with darkening of skin lesions to mauve, slate-grey, or black; red colouration of urine, stools, sputum, sweat and tears; dryness of skin, particularly of forearms and lower legs, which may progress to typical ichthyosis; and, less commonly, irritation or burning discomfort in skin lesions. Gastrointestinal disturbance is usually insignificant at this dosage, especially if clofazimine is taken after food, but patients with light skins find skin pigmentation embarrassing. On p. 99, mention was made of the first report of clofazimine resistance. The drug is safe for the pregnant woman, but more studies of infant mortality will have to be made now that there has been a report of three neonatal deaths in 15 pregnancies.[17] A 15 page booklet on clofazimine has been published by Ciba-Geigy and has been reproduced in *Leprosy Review* (1979); **50**: 135

RIFAMPICIN (RIFAMPIN RFP; RMP; RIFADIN; RIMACTANE)

A semisynthetic derivative of rifamycin B, one of a group of antibiotic compounds produced by *Streptomyces meditteranei*. A forerunner of rifampicin was rifamycin SV, introduced by Opromolla in Brazil in 1963,[18] and early publications on its successor, rifampicin, appeared in 1970. Since then this antibiotic has become established as a highly potent bactericidal drug, and it is likely that its rapid action in killing *M. leprae* is due to inhibition of ribonucleic acid (RNA) synthesis. Rees and his colleagues reported in 1970[19] that it had a rapid action in human leprosy, the morphological index (MI) of bacilli in skin reaching 0 in 5 weeks as against 5 months in control lepromatous cases on dapsone, and they found it effective against dapsone-resistant bacilli. They gave 600 mg daily in a single dose before breakfast, and reduced the daily dose to 450 mg for patients weighing less than 35 kg. No toxic effects were encountered and lepra reaction was a minor problem. Since then the rapid action of rifampicin in rendering bacilli in human skin non-infective to mice has been demonstrated in a number of trials. A dosage of 600 mg daily was able to do this within 14 days in one trial[20] and a similar result was obtained within 5 days in a later trial with a single dose of 1200 mg.[21] The advantages of having an antibiotic that will do this, and at the same time render the patient

The diagram shows one side of the blister calendar pack. The drugs at the top left are given under supervision once-monthly. Those labelled 2–28 are taken by the patient daily, at home, unsupervised. On the other side of the pack, the tablets and capsules are clearly visible in their individual 'bubbles' which are pressed out on administration.

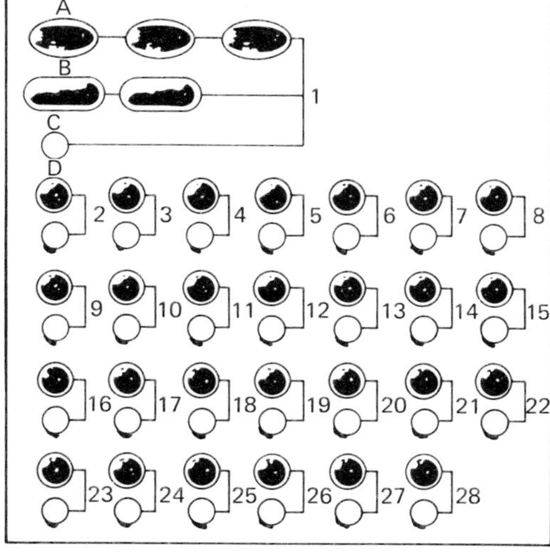

A Clofazimine 100 mg (Lamprene 100 mg capsule)
B Rifampicin 300 mg (Rimactane 300 mg capsule)
C Dapsone 100 mg (Servidapsone 100 mg tablets)
D Clofazimine 50 mg (Lamprene 50 mg capsule)

The leprosy patient receives on day 1 the three drugs illustrated in the diagram at step 1 from his doctor or paramedic.
Afterwards he takes the corresponding medication every day.
On day 29 he goes back to be controlled and to receive a new pack of medication.
In this way the package itself becomes a calendar.

Fig. 8.1 A blister calendar pack for drugs used in treatment of multibacillary leprosy; those at the top left are given under supervision. (Reproduced with kind permission of Ciba-Geigy Ltd from *Leprosy can be Cured*, 1st edn., Basle: Ciba-Geigy, published 1985.)

tuberculosis specialist advises the course which the Medical Research Council has found the most effective: streptomycin, rifampicin, isoniazid and pyrazinamide for the first 2 months, then rifampicin and isoniazid (Medical Research Council 1986 recommendation) for the next 4 months.[38] *For PBL*, nothing need be added during the first 2 months as streptomycin has an acceptable antileprosy action over such a short period, but add dapsone over the last 4 months. *For MBL*, add dapsone during the first 2 months (thus supplying three antileprosy drugs), and then add dapsone and clofazimine during the next 4 months, after which the patient continues on standard multidrug therapy. In view of the number of drugs employed in treating two diseases, the leprologist should take extra care to watch for side-effects, and it would be wise to arrange for regular blood counts and liver function tests. (See Table 8.3 for dosage in children.)

Table 8.3 Guide for drug dosage in children

Dose in relation to adult dose	*Weight range (kg)*
One-quarter	Under 15
One-half	15–30
Three-quarters	30–45
Adult dose	Over 45

REFERENCES

1 Faget G. H., Pogge R. C., Johansen F. A., Dinan J. F., Prejean B. M., Eccles C. G. (1943). The Promin treatment of leprosy: a progress report. *Public Health Reports*; **58**: 1729–41.

2 Seydel J. K., Richter M., Wempe E. (1980). Mechanisms of action of the folate blocker diaminodiphenylsulfone (dapsone, DDS) studied in comparison to sulfonamides (SA). *International Journal of Leprosy*; **48**: 18–29.

3 French T. M. (1968). An injection solution of dapsone. *Leprosy Review*; **39**: 171.

4 Jopling W. H. (1983). Side-effects of antileprosy drugs in common use. *Leprosy Review*; **54**: 261–70.

5 Jopling W. H. (1985). References to 'side-effects of antileprosy drugs in common use'. *Leprosy Review*; **56**: 61–70.

6 Degowin R. L., Eppes R. B., Powell R. D., Carson P. E. (1966). The haemolytic effect of diamino-diphenylsulfone (DDS) in normal subjects and in those with glucose-6-phosphate-dehydrogenase deficiency. *Bulletin of the World Health Organization*; **35**: 165–79.

7 Manfredi G., De Panfilis G., Zampetti M., Allegra F. (1979). Studies on dapsone induced haemolytic anaemia, 1. Methaemoglobin production and G-6-PD activity in correlation with dapsone dosage. *British Journal of Dermatology*; **100**; 427–32.

8 Barss P. (1986). Fatal dapsone agranulocytosis in a Melanesian. *Leprosy Review*; **57**: 63–6.

9 Ognibene A. J. (1970). Agranulocytosis due to dapsone. *Annals of Internal Medicine*; **72**: 521–4.

10 Jopling W. H. (1972). Why agranulocytosis from dapsone? *Annals of Internal Medicine*; **77**: 153.

11 Ackroyd J. F. (1985). Fixed drug eruptions. *British Medical Journal*; **290**: 1533–4.
12 Reigart J. R., Trammel H. L. Jr., Lindsey J. M. (1982–3). Repetitive doses of activated charcoal in dapsone poisoning in a child. *Journal of Toxicology and Clinical Toxicology*; **19**: 1061–6.
13 Huikeshoven H., Baller J., Agusni I. *et al.* (1984). Multi-centre evaluation of a spot test for detection of dapsone in urine. *Abstracts of XII International Leprosy Congress*; No. IX/374(A).
14 Huikeshoven H. (1984). Multi-centre evaluation of a spot test for detection of dapsone in urine. *The STAR*; **43**: 12–13.
15 Huikeshoven H., Madarang M. G. (1986). Spot test for detection of dapsone in urine: an assessment of its validity and interpretation. *International Journal of Leprosy*; **54**: 21–4.
16 Browne S. G., Hogerzeil L. M. (1962). 'B 663' in the treatment of leprosy: preliminary report of a pilot trial. *Leprosy Review*; **33**: 6–10.
17 Farb H., West D. P., Pedvis–Leftick A. (1982). Clofazimine in pregnancy complicated by leprosy. *Obstetrics and Gynaecology*; **59**: 122–3.
18 Opromolla D. V. A. (1963). First results of the use of Rifamycin SV in the treatment of lepromatous leprosy. *International Journal of Leprosy*; **31**: 552.
19 Rees R. J. W., Pearson J. M. H., Waters M. F. R. (1970). Experimental and clinical studies on rifampicin in treatment of leprosy. *British Medical Journal*; **1**: 89–92.
20 Shepard C. C., Levy L., Fasal P. (1976). Further experience with the rapid bactericidal effect of rifampin on *Mycobacterium leprae* in man. *American Journal of Tropical Medicine & Hygiene*; **23**: 1120–4.
21 Levy L., Shepard C. C., Fasal P. (1976). The bactericidal effect of rifampicin on *M. Leprae* in man: a) single doses of 600, 900 and 1200 mg; and b) daily doses of 300 mg. *International Journal of Leprosy*; **44**: 183–7.
22 Rees R. J. W., Waters M. F. R., Pearson J. M. H., Helmy H. S., Laing A. B. G. (1976). Long-term treatment of dapsone-resistant leprosy with rifampicin: clinical and bacteriological studies. *International Journal of Leprosy*; **44**: 159–69.
23 Opromolla D. V. A., Tonello C. J. S., McDougall A. C.,

Yawalkar S. J. (1981). A controlled trial to compare the therapeutic effects of dapsone in combination with daily or once-monthly rifampicin in patients with lepromatous leprosy. *International Journal of Leprosy*; **49**: 393–7.

24 Gill G. V. (1976). Rifampicin and breakfast. *Lancet*; **ii**: 1135.

25 Wise R. (1987). Prescribing in pregnancy: antibiotics. *British Medical Journal*; **294**: 42–6.

26 Jopling W. H., Pettit J. H. S. (1979). Interaction between rifampicin, steroids and oral contraceptives. *Leprosy Review*; **50**: 331–2.

27 McAllister W. A. C., Thompson P. J., Al-Habet S. M., Rogers H. J. (1983). Rifampicin reduces effectiveness and bioavailability of prednisone. *British Medical Journal*; **286**: 923–5.

28 Jacobson R. R., Hastings R. C. (1976). Rifampin-resistant leprosy. *Lancet*; **ii**: 1304–5.

29 Colston M. J., Hilson G. R. F., Lancaster R. D. (1980). The effect of intermittent ethionamide and combinations of ethionamide and dapsone in experimental leprosy in mice. In *Leprosy. Proceedings of the XI International Leprosy Congress*, Mexico City, November 13–18 (1978) (Latapi F. *et al.*, eds). Amsterdam, Oxford, Princeton: Excerpta Medica.

30 Shepard C. C. (1972). Combinations of drugs against *Mycobactrium leprae* studied in mice. *International Journal of Leprosy*; **40**: 33–9.

31 World Health Organization Study Group. (1982). *Chemotherapy of Leprosy* for *Control Programmes*. Technical Report Series No. 657. Geneva: WHO.

32 Freerksen E., Rosenfeld M. (1977). Leprosy eradication project of Malta. *Chemotherapy*; **23**: 356–86.

33 Jopling W. H., Ridley M. J., Bonnici E., Depasquale G. (1984). A follow-up investigation of the Malta-Project. *Leprosy Review*; **55**: 247–53.

34 Jopling W. H. (1986). A report on two follow-up investigations of the Malta-Project. *Leprosy Review*; **57**: 47–52.

35 Winsley B. E., McDougall A. C., Brown K. E. (1983). Chemotherapy of leprosy: 'bubble' or 'calendar' packs for the administration of rifampin, dapsone, clofazimine or prothionamide/ethionamide. *International Journal of Leprosy*; **51**: 592–4.

36 Wiseman L. A. (1987). Calendar (blister) packs for multidrug

therapy in leprosy: an inexpensive, locally-produced version. *Leprosy Review*; **58**: 85–7.

37 Georgiev G. D., Kielstrup R. W. (1987). Blister calendar packs for the implementation of multiple drug therapy in DANIDA – assisted leprosy control projects in India. *Leprosy Review*; **58**: 249–55.

38 East and Central African/British Medical Research Council Fifth Collaborative Study. (1986). Controlled clinical trial of 4 short-course regimens of chemotherapy (three 6-month and one 8-month) for pulmonary tuberculosis: final report. *Tubercle*; **67**: 5–15.

9 Other Aspects of Treatment

1. MANAGEMENT OF LEPRA REACTION

The management of Type 1 reaction is the management of neuritis, and this will be found below.

Problems in Type 2 reaction are multiple, as many organs and tissues can be involved in the immune complex syndrome. First of all the possibility of an intercurrent infection must be excluded, and a thought should be given to the other causes of Type 2 reaction mentioned in Chapter 6. The patient will require assurance, as his first assumption will be that his leprosy has taken a turn for the worse. He can be told that the reverse holds good, for the reaction is a sign that his leprosy bacilli are being killed. However, in spite of reassurance he may need a tranquilliser, for worrying about his reaction is a sure way of aggravating it. He may need an analgesic to relieve pain in bones or joints (nerve pain is dealt with in a separate section below). ENL lesions may respond to a few injections of a trivalent antimony compound. Above all, bed rest should be avoided as it encourages boredom, introspection and mental depression; it is better to keep the patient active and on light duties. Anti-inflammatory agents, such as indomethacin (Indocid) and flufenamic acid (Arlef) can be tried, but their effect is unreliable and large doses cause unpleasant side-effects. Aspirin is as good as any. The authors have found chloroquine valueless.

When the reaction is more severe, with fever, prostration, extensive ENL, severe pain and other manifestations, the two drugs of proven value are prednisone (prednisolone) and thalidomide.

Steroid (corticosteroids)

Steroid therapy is a well-established method of controlling the worst aspects of lepra reaction: neuritis in Type 1 reaction (the only serious manifestation of this type of reaction), and, in Type 2

nerve function. Suitable supportive therapy for paralysed muscles is required in the form of padded splints, and sessions of graduated exercises and active exercises will aid muscle recovery and prevent stiffness in joints.[5] The authors have seen complete recovery of sensory and motor paralysis occurring in upgrading reactions in borderline leprosy, aided by prednisone, without interrupting antileprosy therapy.

Although it might be argued that adrenocorticotrophic hormone (ATCH) injections are preferable to prednisone because they act by stimulating the patient's adrenal cortex to produce extra cortisol, thus avoiding adrenocortical atrophy, their effect in lepra reaction is slower and less reliable. Furthermore, they can depress anterior pituitary function. ATCH injections can be given intramuscularly as the gel in daily doses of 40 units at first, gradually increasing the interval between injections to every other day and then to twice a week, after which the strength of each injection can be reduced.

Intraneural injections

These can be given for the relief of severe nerve pain. One method is to draw up 1 ml of 2% lignocaine into a syringe, dissolve 1500 units of hyaluronidase (Hyalase) in it, and then draw up 1 ml of hydrocortisone suspension (25 mg/ml). This is slowly injected into the swollen nerve, or around it, using a size 14 needle after infiltrating the skin with local anaesthetic.

Surgical treatment

A number of papers have described the role of surgery in the treatment of chronic neuritis in leprosy, particularly when affecting the ulnar nerve, and references are given in a paper by Palande.[6] These papers establish the value of neurolysis and of nerve transposition in relieving pain and improving nerve function so long as there is proper selection of cases. The word 'neurolysis' implies surgical decompression either by incising the nerve sheath or by excising it. However, experienced surgeons admit that the need for nerve surgery has declined in centres where anti-inflammatory drugs such as prednisone, thalidomide and clofazimine are available and are correctly used.[7] Cubital tunnel external compression syndrome can be mimicked by ulnar nerve neuritis in leprosy, and orthopaedic surgeons working in countries like Britain where leprosy is not endemic may miss the true diagnosis unless they think of leprosy and question the patient about past residence in the tropics. Surgical transposition of the ulnar nerve[8] is unlikely to be of value in leprosy, as pathological changes are within the nerve. But, if the nerve is subject to repeated trauma this operation will benefit a small minority. It has been proposed[9] that this minority can be selected by: (1) the presence of a small interval between the olecranon and the medial epicondyle of the humerus (25 mm or less with the elbow extended); (2) increase of this interval by more than 50% with the elbow fully flexed. Surgical evacuation is required for a nerve abscess and the wound can be closed without drainage.

Acute iritis (iridocyclitis)

This calls for *hourly* instillation of steroid eyedrops such as 1% cortisone or hydrocortisone by day (this intensive treatment is reserved for the acute stage, after which the drops are instilled b.d.) and the application of a steroid eye ointment such as 2% cortisone at night. Eyedrops of 1% homatropine or of 1% cyclopentolate (Mydrilate) must be instilled twice a day in an attempt to keep the pupil as dilated as possible and so prevent or counter adhesions (synechiae). This treatment should be continued after the acute phase has subsided, and a slit-lamp is of great value in deciding if and when the cellular exudate disappears from the aqueous humour. Fortunately, glaucoma is a rare complication in leprosy, but if it is suspected because of increase in eyeball pain and tension, acetazolamide (Diamox) should be given in dosage of 250 mg two or three times a day. This acts by interfering with the production of aqueous humour. It would also be wise to give oral steroid in addition (see above for dosage). In patients whose eyes have been neglected or incorrectly treated, and posterior synechiae have formed a complete ring round the pupil, Choyce[10] advocates a complete iridectomy; this prevents secondary glaucoma from iris bombé, delays the onset of complicated cataract, and attacks of acute iridocyclitis become less troublesome.

Acute epididymo-orchitis

This needs prompt treatment with prednisone and the scrotum should be supported by a suspensory bandage (Fig. 9.2).

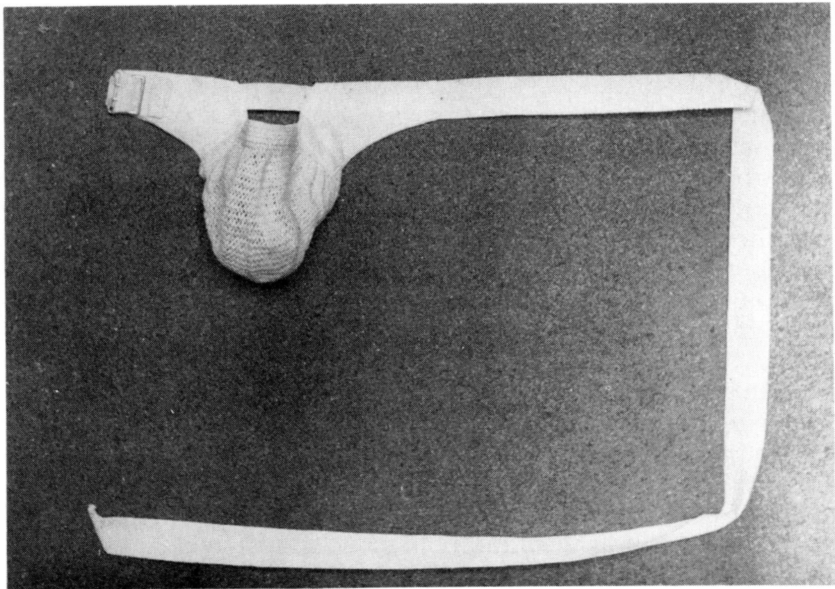

Fig. 9.2 A suspensory bandage.

2. CARE OF HANDS AND FEET

This is a very important aspect of management, as the anaesthetic hand or foot is repeatedly injured by the careless patient, and because of the absence of pain the injured limb is not rested and healing is therefore protracted and often complicated by sepsis. This gives the false impression that the leprosy patient has an impaired healing capacity. On the question of the best dressing to apply for plantar ulcer, each clinician will draw on his own experience, but in general it is advisable to avoid ointments or powders containing antibiotics because of the risk of sensitisation. The authors recommend Anaflex ointment or powder, as polynoxylin is not an antibiotic, does not sensitise and is a very reliable antibacterial substance. Chronic plantar ulceration is a more important cause of morbidity, impaired working capacity and loss of working time, than is leprosy itself, for it continues to be a problem long after the leprosy has been arrested – in fact, for the rest of the patient's life. A chiropodist can play a very important role in both the prevention and treatment of plantar ulceration, and should be considered an essential member of the medical team.[11] Together with injuries to hands, plantar ulceration is a particularly common complication of lepromatous leprosy, for the arrest of the disease is associated with progressive fibrosis of nerves resulting in 'glove and stocking' anaesthesia and intrinsic muscle weakness is late to develop. The care of hands and feet involves the education of the patient on how to care for his limbs, the avoidance of burns of the hands, the wearing of correct footwear, the regular daily examination of hands and feet for minor injuries (which would otherwise go unobserved), and the prompt treatment of any injuries found. The likelihood of burns to the hands can be reduced by wearing suitable gloves when cooking or attending to fires, by giving up cigarette smoking or by using a cigarette holder, and by insulating the handles of all cooking utensils so that they do not conduct heat. Insensitive legs can be burned by sitting too close to a fire or heater, or by the use of a hot-water bottle in bed.

To avoid plantar ulceration the patient must avoid all unnecessary standing and walking, all hurrying or running, must learn to take short steps and should soften the callosities which form under the heads of the metatarsals by soaking the feet in warm water daily for 10–15 minutes. Then the callosities are rubbed with pumice or with a callus file as made by Scholl and retailed by most chemists. The patient must wear suitable footwear *throughout the day* – in the house as well as out of doors. A sandal with a strong stiff sole is ideal in the tropics, and it should be lined by a Plastazote insole[12,13] which is glued in position to prevent shifting. Alternatively, insoles can be made of microcellular rubber.[14] If shoes are worn they should be strong, comfortable, free from nails, broad at the toes and without toecap, and, as with sandals, should be worn throughout the day. Ideally they should be made to measure, the tongues should be of extra width, the sole should be of stiff leather, and laces should be avoided if the patient has deformed fingers, in which case Velcro is the ideal alternative. Slippers and rubber-soled shoes such as tennis shoes should never be worn. The patient must be advised about 'wearing-in' new shoes before they can be worn all day, and this means wearing them for an hour a day during the first week, 2 hours a day for the second week, and so on. Shoes that are being regularly worn and have become moulded to the shape of the feet should be ranked among the patient's most treasured possessions and can be repeatedly resoled until they literally drop to pieces. Plastazote insoles can play an important part in the prevention of plantar ulceration,[15] as they are moulded to the shape of each sole, and it is even possible to have shoes made entirely of this material. Plastazote has been marketed by Smith & Nephew Pharmaceuticals Limited, Bessemer Road, Welwyn Garden City, Herts., England.

An alternative to a Plastazote insole is to make use of the Harris footprint mat to demonstrate the areas of the sole receiving abnormal pressure on standing or walking. (Obtainable from Messrs. Heinrich Ad. Berkemann, PO Box 540740, D-2 Hamburg 54, West Germany.) The insole can then be suitably moulded in order to distribute weight-bearing over the areas of skin which are not doing their fair share. The Harris footprint mat is made of rubber and consists of thousands of ridges of three different heights; the mat is inked, and a piece of paper is placed over it. When a person stands or steps on it, the amount of pressure each small area of foot carries can be determined.

Once an ulcer has formed, an attempt can be made to heal it by the general measures described above. However, if these fail, the ulcer can be healed by bed rest (crutches are useful to ensure 100% avoidance of weight bearing) and adhesive zinc tape is the dressing of choice for the ulcer.[16] The alternative is a below-knee walking plaster maintained for about 5 weeks. A useful method of reducing the likelihood of the insensitive leg becoming abraded by the plaster is to cover the foot and leg with a crepe bandage before applying the plaster of Paris. It is essential, if recurrence of plantar ulceration is to be avoided, to supply suitable footwear once the plaster has been removed; if this is neglected a recurrence rate of 40% can be expected.[17] If the ulcer is complicated by cellulitis, a swab is taken for culture and sensitivity tests, and a broad spectrum antibiotic is prescribed pending the result of sensitivity testing. A radiograph is necessary in order to assess the condition of the bones of the foot. The problem of foot care in leprosy has been discussed by Brand,[18] and Grace Warren[19] has stressed the importance of treating tarsal bone disintegration by immobilising the foot in a walking plaster for a minimum period of 5 months.

Physiotherapy is important to keep fingers mobile and to prevent contractures[5] and in its simplest form means teaching the patient to carry out simple exercises daily; these should include extending paralysed fingers to their fullest extent by pressing the dorsal surfaces of the first phalanges against the thigh, which makes it easier to extend them, and massaging them while in this position. A well-padded splint, which extends the fingers by pressing on the dorsa of the first phalanges, can be worn at night. Namasivayan has devised a simple method of keeping paralysed fingers extended when the hand is not in use,[20] thus protecting paralysed intrinsic muscles from stretching while in a stage of recovery and preventing flexion contracture at the first interphalangeal joint. He uses a galvanised iron wire of 8 or 10 gauge, about 29 cm long, inserted into rubber tubing with an internal diameter of 2–3 mm and about 30 cm long, bent to form an 'S'-shaped spiral (Figs. 9.3a, b and c).

Electroacupuncture produces electric impulses similar to nerve impulses, and can give active exercise to completely paralysed muscles, thus preventing disuse atrophy of these muscles.[21]

3. CHRONIC LEG ULCERATION

This can arise in an insensitive leg either from a breaking down leprosy lesion, from a group of necrotic ENL lesions, or from a neglected abrasion. If it is allowed to persist for years it can lead to secondary amyloidosis or to malignant changes in the ulcer. Its management differs from that of a plantar ulcer in that it is not subjected to repeated trauma, and three lines of treatment are worth considering, used singly or in combination, before having recourse to skin grafting.

1. Granuflex (Squibb) – flexible hydroactive dressings. The authors recommend this line of treatment using dressings of 100 mm^2 size or of 200 mm^2 size, depending on the size of the ulcer, and dressings can be changed every week. There should be no interference with the bed of the ulcer (however good the intentions may be) apart from a saline irrigation before each change of dressing.
2. Local applications of adhesive zinc tape have given good results in India, with the advantage of cheapness, ease of application and avoidance of bandages.[22]
3. Levamisole by mouth has been shown to have a dramatic effect in healing chronic leg ulceration from various causes.[23]

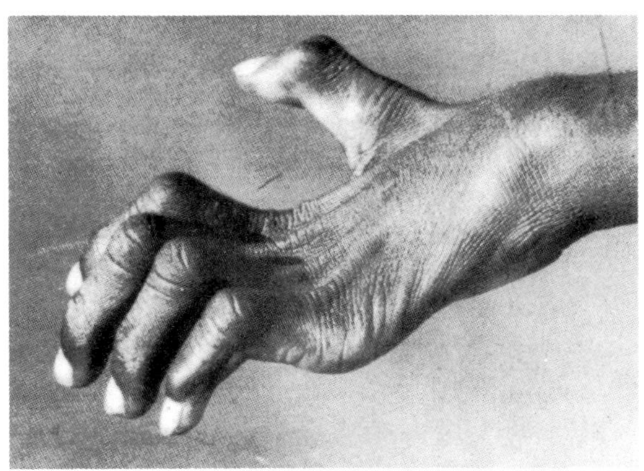

(a)

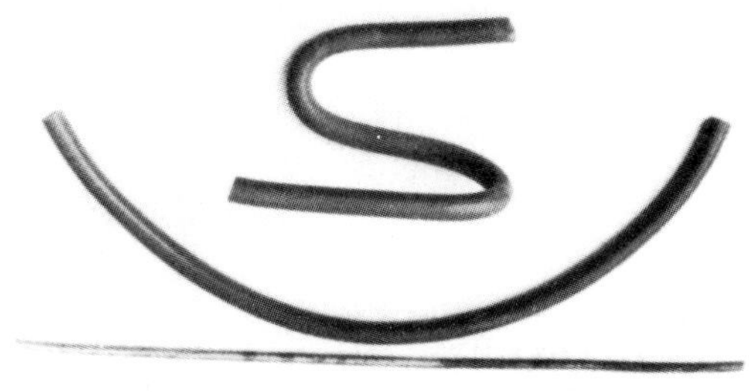

(b)

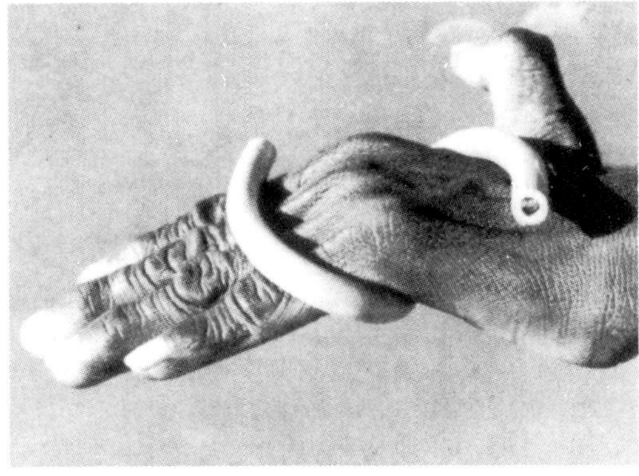

(c)

Fig. 9.3a, b and c **a** = Intrinsic muscle paralysis of the hand. The fact that the fingers can be extended passively can be seen in b and c showing the same hand in a Namasivayan's splint. **b** = Hand splint – galvanised iron wire inserted into rubber tubing. **c** = Hand splint in position. (Figs. 9.3b and c reproduced by kind permission of the editor of *Leprosy in India.*)

Its potential in treating patients who are immunodepressed or immunodeficient has been discussed on p. 79. Its effect in treating leg ulceration in leprosy has yet to be determined. Amery and Morias[23] gave a dose of 2·5 mg/kg on 2 consecutive days each week over a 20-week period.

4. MANAGEMENT OF LEPROUS RHINITIS

Barton[24] has given full details, and he stresses the risk of trauma to the nasal septum, resulting in ulceration, if the patient attempts to remove crusts by 'picking' his nose, especially as over one-half of the patients examined for leprous atrophic rhinitis are likely to have some degree of sensory loss in the nose. Removal of crusts by means of nasal dressings forceps is best done at the leprosy clinic, and adherent crusts can be softened by irrigation with a solution containing 5 g each of sodium bicarbonate, sodium borate and sodium chloride, dissolved in 500 ml of warm water. After removal of crusts, the nasal cavities are liberally smeared with an ointment made up as follows:[25] Vaseline 100 g, glycerine 20 g and Vioform 30 g. Vioform is the trade name of clioquinol, the ingredient of Entero-Vioform tablets. In the event of Vioform being withdrawn from the market[25] the best substitute would be Anaflex powder, in the same proportion. The ointment is applied on cotton-wool-tipped sticks which can either be made in the clinic or can be bought in the form of 'cotton buds' (Johnson and Johnson), or 'Q-tips' (Chesebrough-Ponds) as used in baby care.

Epistaxis can be controlled by inserting a piece of 'Sterispon' (A & H) absorbable gelatin sponge.

5. CARE OF THE EYES

Eyes should be regularly examined, and the importance of looking for 'insidious iritis' in lepromatous leprosy has been mentioned in Chapter 2; the patient has no ocular discomfort or redness, and the only means of detecting this insidious condition is by means of the corneal microscope (slit lamp). The treatment of acute iritis has been described in the section on 'Management of Lepra Reaction' (p. 126). Patients with early lagophthalmos must be encouraged to exercise the eyelids by frequent forced closure, and a tear substitute such as 0·5% methyl cellulose or castor oil is required for those with more advanced lagophthalmos in order to prevent drying of the conjunctiva. The wearing of an eye shield, especially when lagophthalmos is associated with corneal anaesthesia, is of proven value.[26] When the lower lid is completely paralysed and there is danger of exposure keratitis, a lateral tarsorrhaphy is a simple operation designed to unite the eyelids at their lateral aspect; temporalis transfer, a more complicated operation, involves the use of a fascial sling attached to a slip of temporalis muscle which by active contraction (clenching the teeth) closes the lids.

All who are responsible for the care of leprosy patients should study Margaret Brand's pamphlet *The Care of the Eye in Hansen's Disease* (see Table 6.2, p. 89).

6. ORTHOPAEDIC AND PLASTIC SURGERY

Surgery has an important part to play in the rehabilitation of the leprosy patient. Paralysed fingers, so long as they are not ankylosed, can be straightened by the many-tailed graft of Brand using plantaris tendon, dropped foot can be corrected by transfer of tibialis posterior muscle preceded, if the foot is unstable, by triple arthrodesis, and clawed fingers or toes can be corrected. Because of the ever-present problem of anaesthesia, causing the patient to be careless, *hand and foot surgery in leprosy should be judged, not by its technical perfection, but by its long-term results*. Plastic surgery is required for gynaecomastia, facial palsy, nasal deformity, loss of eyebrows, lagophthalmos, and facial disfigurement due to excessive folds of skin. Operative details can be found in a number of publications. When chronic plantar ulceration has not responded to conservative methods, the removal of a damaged or infected metatarsal, combined with excision of the ulcer, may provide a permanent cure.

Gross deformity or bone infection will require below-knee amputation; Syme's amputation is unsatisfactory in leprosy because of ulceration developing in the insensitive heel-flap. As the stump in a below-knee amputation is likely to be insensitive, wearing an artificial limb may cause ulceration of the stump; a lining of Plastazote can protect the skin from trauma. Where surgical treatment for dropped foot is not considered suitable, the patient can be supplied with a toespring support fixed to his shoe.

The tendency to hypoprothrombinaemia in LL patients (see p.

21), as shown by increased prothrombin and clotting times, is a potential hazard in major surgery. A patient found to have a prolonged prothrombin time prior to surgery can be given an intravenous injection of Dried Factor IX Fraction (BP) or of Factor IX Complex (USP). These preparations contain coagulation fractions II, IX and X, obtained from human plasma.

7. OTHER TREATMENT

Dry skin

This is commonly experienced in long-standing LL and usually affects arms and legs bilaterally. Dry skin is due to lack of sweating which, in turn, is due to failure of autonomic fibres within damaged dermal nerves to stimulate sweat glands. Mild degrees of dry skin respond to daily soaking for about 15 minutes in warm water, followed by application of white soft paraffin (white petroleum jelly BP) to the affected regions of skin, in order to occlude water loss from the outer layer of skin. In the tropics, where a minimum of clothes are worn, the emollient can be rubbed into the wet skin, but in temperate regions it is applied to the damp skin after light towelling. Severe degrees of dryness (ichthyosis), commonly associated with clofazimine treatment, respond better to a cream containing 10% carbamide (urea), the main constituent of Calmurid and Aquadrate, applied to damp skin. When eczema complicates dry skin, as it often does in leprosy, a useful cream is one which combines 10% urea with 1% hydrocortisone (Calmurid HC; Alphaderm).

Breast pain

This may occur in males who are developing gynaecomastia, and is due to testosterone–oestrogen imbalance, i.e. normal oestrogen production by the adrenal cortex and deficient testosterone production by the damaged testes. It can be relieved by testosterone injections (see below).

Impotence

This is a common late complication of lepromatous leprosy, especially if the disease was in an advanced stage when antileprosy

financial support for periods in the order of 3–5 years, a constant supply of the antileprosy drugs needed for both adults and children, laboratory facilities and a system for the referral, and expert treatment of problem cases. Some of these conditions are relatively easy to establish, others extremely difficult. Very few programmes can say that all activities under the main headings 1–4 above have been satisfactorily organised, and in practice the majority need help at almost every level.

It is beyond the scope of this chapter to deal with the whole subject of leprosy control, and from the list of activities which call for attention if a programme is to be successful, the authors select three which have not been fully described in recent publications and which they believe to be of particular importance: (1) analysis, clarification and definition of the total 'prevalence', (2) the supply of drugs for multiple drug therapy, and (3) the prevention and treatment of disability and deformity.

1. Analysis, clarification and definition of the total 'prevalence'

The term 'prevalence', usually taken to mean the number of registered cases in a defined population at a specified time, has come in for a considerable amount of criticism, and because of inherent inaccuracies, most of them to do with the way in which data are collected. Attention has been drawn to the greater importance of incidence or case detection rates in the assessment of the true state of affairs and much scorn has been poured on prevalence figures as misleading and meaningless accumulations of names in a book. But the fact remains that these figures are closely related to the workload, the number of staff employed, the miles travelled and the year-in year-out cost of the programme. One of the authors' medical students recently took a year off to work in a leprosy control programme in Africa. At the outset he was told that there were about 3000 registered patients. On careful examination of the treatment registers during the next few months, neither he (nor the leprosy staff) were able to record more than 2200. He then deducted those who were dead or had left the region or the country, double (and some treble) entries, together with those who had neither attended nor had been heard of for 2 years or more. The figure was now well under 2000. Although he lacked the experience or ability to proceed further, his impression was that *only about one-half* of those remaining needed any form of chemotherapy or further medical care. Critical analysis and up-dating of leprosy patient registers should be carried out at least once-yearly in every programme. The process is outstandingly important *before* starting a programme using multiple drug therapy. Indeed, there is now much evidence from various parts of the world that a determined analysis of all patients *before implementing such therapy* has often produced reductions in 'prevalence' in the order of 25–30%.

2. The supply of drugs for multiple drug therapy

It is not infrequently stated, with considerable justification, that multiple drug therapy, involving drugs such as dapsone, rifampicin, clofazimine and possibly prothionamide/ethionamide, should not be considered unless the health staff is adequate in numbers and standards of performance. Unfortunately, it is difficult to define these standards in a useful manner and to list the conditions which render implementation reasonable and safe on the one hand, or unacceptable and potentially dangerous on the other. In a previous publication,[4] an attempt was made to list the characteristics of satisfactory and unsatisfactory levels of performance, and these may give some indication of programmes in which multiple drug therapy can be implemented or not. Most programmes, however, probably lie between these two extremes and in them it is therefore particularly important to examine the various factors which impede MDT implementation. Why is it, in late 1987, 5 full years after the publication of the WHO recommendations on MDT, that only 8% of all registered cases in the world are on MDT?

Of the many factors which may be concerned, one which merits further study is the ordering, purchase, central supply, despatch and storage of the drugs needed, together with their dispensing by health staff and use by patients. Very little expert attention has been given to this complex but important process. Experience through the decades, even with dapsone as monotherapy, shows clearly that the chain of events is likely to falter at almost every stage. Programme managers frequently fail to order adequate quantities well in advance. Ministries of health and central pharmacies have difficulty in ordering and stocking all the drugs (in adult and child denominations) needed for MDT in peripheral units, which are directly responsible for the issue of drugs to patients on a regular and systematic basis. They often find that deliveries are either late or incomplete. If MDT is attempted, *all* the drugs must be available on a dependable and regular basis from start to finish.

One potentially useful device in this context, which has attracted increasing attention in recent years, is the 'blister' calendar pack (see p. 115) for the dispensing of drugs to both pauci- and multibacillary patients. Experience in their use over the past 2 years in the Philippines[5] and more recently in India[6,7] has shown that they are extremely popular with health staff and patients. The dispensing of drugs in blister packs may add up to 15% to the total cost of medication, but their cost-effectiveness and potential in facilitating the implementation of MDT and possibly in improving compliance and regularity of attendance should not be underestimated. A trial to compare the value of blister packs versus the handling and dispensing of drugs 'loose' is currently under way in Thailand.[8] Preliminary impressions from these three different countries indicate that blister packs may also be of positive value in (1) preserving antileprosy drugs in good condition after dispensing to patients, (2) reducing misuse and pilfering, and (3) enhancing the status of the medication offered for treatment of this disease, and (4) facilitating the work of health staff.

3. The prevention and treatment of disability and deformity

Those who have first-hand knowledge of leprosy often claim, that although the skin lesions are unsightly and at times alarming, they are rarely of long-term significance because they normally respond to treatment and disappear, often in a matter of months. Nerve damage, however, especially if established at the outset before effective treatment is another matter. By no means all damage to sensory and motor fibres is reversible; much of it is permanent leading to paralysis and sensory loss. If there is one thing better than the treatment of deformity and disability in leprosy it is, of course, prevention, and the authors feel that disability prevention should be given a much higher priority in the control programme than has been the case in recent years. Case detection and chemotherapy are of course fundamental, but the programme will be considered to have failed, not only by the patients but also by the health staff and the general public, if something effective is not done about disability. Jean Watson of The Leprosy Mission International in London has proposed that leprosy control should be divided, perhaps about equally, between '*bacillus control*' and '*disability control*'. Both might be under the technical guidance of a medically qualified programme manager (if one is available) but it is thought that *disability control* should be organised by an experienced national physiotherapist, with responsibility for health education, training of staff and the provision of workshops, and other facilities for protective footwear and prostheses.

We all look forward towards eradication. Meanwhile it would be an advance if the majority of leprosy-endemic countries could either eliminate the disease as a significant public health problem or bring it down to a level at which the general health services can safely and effectively cope with new or remaining cases. In many parts of the world, however, there is so much to be done before these stages are reached that we return, by way of emphasis, to the concept of improvement. It is not beyond us to construct sound plans of action; train our staff to reasonable levels of competence; define the problem in terms of patients actually needing MDT; ensure that drug supplies are available; prevent and treat disability. All this calls for perseverence. We must avoid grandiose schemes and concentrate on what Blake called the 'minute particulars'.[9] It may well be that our chances of advancing towards the eradication of leprosy are better now than they have ever been before.

REFERENCES

1 World Health Organization (1982). *Chemotherapy of Leprosy for Control Programmes*. Report of WHO Study Group. Technical Report Series 675. Geneva: WHO.

2 World Health Organization (1985). *Epidemiology of Leprosy in Relation to Control*. Report of WHO Study Group. Technical Report Series 716. Geneva: WHO.

3 World Health Organization (1987). *Report of the Second Coordinating Meeting on the Implementation of Multidrug Therapy in*

Leprosy Control Programmes. WHO/CDS/LEP 87.2. Limited distribution. Geneva: WHO.
4 McDougall A. C. (1982). Editorial. *International Journal of Leprosy*; **50**: 355–8.
5 Yuasa Y. (1987). Personal communication.
6 Revankar C. R., Sørensen B. H. (1988). Letter to the editor. *Leprosy Review*; **59**: in press.
7 Georgiev G. D., Kielstrup R. W. (1987). Blister calendar packs for the implementation of multiple drug therapy in DANIDA – assisted leprosy control projects in India. *Leprosy Review*; **58**: 249–55.
8 McDougall A. C. (1987). Protocol for a controlled clinical trial of blister-calendar packs for the treatment of leprosy with multiple drug therapy (MDT) in Thailand. (Unpublished document.)
9 Woodruff A. W., Adamson E. A., El Suni A., Maughan T. S., Kaku M., Bundru W. (1986). Children in Juba, southern Sudan: the second and third years of life. *Lancet*; **ii**: 615–18.

11 Prevention

The basic factors in the prevention of leprosy in endemic regions are:

1 case-finding and prompt treatment of all cases found,
2 keeping the families of patients under surveillance and giving immunoprophylaxis to lepromin-negative contacts,
3 giving BCG vaccination (or an improved vaccine when it becomes available) to all young children, particularly to all infants newly born into leprous families.
4 improvement in living conditions, especially housing, so that members of families do not have to live in close contact,
5 education and propaganda about leprosy.

In the presulphone era, compulsory segregation of leprosy sufferers was the only public health measure which was applicable. Its objective was to isolate the sources of infection, but its value was limited because those with early and active disease (the infectious cases) hid the fact in order to avoid being forcibly removed from their homes. This has been seen in the failure of compulsory segregation to control the disease in the many tropical countries which attempted this method of control. It would be a mistake to give segregation the credit for the decline of leprosy in Norway in the latter part of the 19th century, for two main reasons. First, segregation in Norway was based on the assumption that leprosy was hereditary and that sexual isolation of the patients would prevent them from passing on the disease;[1] inmates of the leprosy hospital in Bergen were allowed to go to the market to sell the wares that they had made. Second, tuberculosis had been endemic in Norway long enough for genetic immunity to tuberculosis to reach maximal proportions by the end of the 19th century, thus providing a degree of cross-immunity to leprosy. In contrast, the epidemiological curve of tuberculosis in most parts of the tropics has not yet begun to descend.

Nowadays, with effective antileprosy drugs, treatment can do what segregation did in the past, and can do it more effectively, more cheaply, and much more pleasantly. Hence the importance of case-finding programmes and of keeping family contacts under review. There is a strong body of opinion that a leprosy control programme should be part of a general public health campaign for that particular region, combining it with the control of tuberculosis and other infectious diseases. However, this view may have to be revised now that we are faced with an increasing problem of dapsone resistance, which will need the undivided attention of the leprosy team if it is to be controlled.

To test the hypothesis that tuberculosis provides cross-immunity to leprosy, and in the absence of a specific leprosy vaccine, trials of BCG vaccination have been carried out in many parts of the world. Three which have received wide publicity are those in East Africa, New Guinea and Burma. The trial in East Africa, involving children, resulted in a reduction of incidence of 80% attributable to BCG vaccination,[2] and the one in Karimui (New Guinea) involving about 5000 persons of all ages, indicated that the efficiency of the programme was 46% for the total population.[2] The trial in Burma, concerned with a child population, showed no difference in leprosy incidence between the vaccinated and unvaccinated groups. Yet, in the group aged 0–4 at intake, BCG-vaccinated children had a protection rate of 44·2%.[2]

It should be noted that laboratory research lends support to the theory of cross-immunity between tuberculosis and leprosy, for BCG vaccination of mice inhibits subsequent multiplication of *M. leprae* in foot pads.[3] It is of more than historical interest that Hansen, in the years following his discovery of the leprosy bacillus, made repeated attempts to infect himself with material obtained from his patients' nodules, with no success. The reason for his failure could be attributed to his immunity to tuberculosis for a few years previously his wife had died of pulmonary tuberculosis and yet he remained healthy. Furthermore, he persuaded his father-in-law, Dr Danielssen, to be inoculated with leprosy bacilli, and the result was equally negative. Danielssen had submitted to the experiment convinced that it would fail because of his deep-rooted conviction that leprosy was a hereditary familial disease; little did he suspect that another mycobacterial disease could have protected him – his attack of pulmonary tuberculosis at 17.

Case-finding is an essential part of any leprosy control programme, and the two most important routine methods are regular examinations of household contacts and of children at school. There are many reports of the value of systematic school medical examinations, and these stress two observations of special interest; first, that early lesions commonly affect skin areas such as back, buttocks and thighs, therefore all clothes must be removed if they are not to be missed; second, the great majority of these children have non-lepromatous leprosy.

As regards education and propaganda about leprosy, the first objective should be to have an informed medical profession so as to reduce delays in diagnosis to a minimum. This involves teaching medical students about the disease and keeping doctors aware of the subject by means of films such as that produced by LEPRA. This film, entitled 'Leprosy', can be bought by hospitals outside Britain on application to the Central Office of Information, Film Division, Hercules Road, London SE1 7DU. Another film has been produced in Germany in collaboration with WHO; it is available in English, German, French and Spanish, and can be obtained from Science Services Berlin, 1000 Berlin 21, Thomasiusstrasse 11, Germany. A more recent film entitled 'The Misunderstood Disease' is a production of the Katharina Kasper Leprosy Control Scheme in India. For details of cost and posting, apply to Project Officer, Leprosy Control Scheme, 38/4 Davis Road, Bangalore 560 005, India. Such films are also of value in the training of nurses and in supplying information about leprosy to schools, universities and to the lay public in general. Doctors who have the task of training medical assistants may like to know that a teaching set of colour transparencies, together with text, can be obtained at low cost from Teaching Aids at Low Cost, c/o The Institute of Child Health, 30 Guildford Street, London WC1N 1EH. The teaching set is entitled 'The Classification of Leprosy'. Another set, 'Leprosy in Childhood', is also available. Recently, the Department of Medical Illustration in Oxford has produced a 14-minute video tape (VHS PAL 625 system) on 'Chemotherapy of Leprosy for Control Programmes'. (Apply to: Department of Medical Illustration, John Radcliffe Hospital, Headington, Oxford OX3 9DU.) The American Leprosy Missions has also produced two slide – script and tape set of 'Leprosy in General Practice' and 'Differential Diagnosis of Leprosy'. (Apply to: American Leprosy Missions, One Broadway, Elmwood Park, New Jersey 07407, USA.)

In Chapter 5 the possibility of making a specific vaccine is discussed, now that adequate supplies of *M. leprae* can be supplied from infected armadillos, but there is serious doubt that it will be effective used alone. However, it is reasonable to hope that combining it with BCG or other suitable mycobacterium may enhance its efficacy.

There is serious doubt regarding the prophylactic use of dapsone or other antileprosy drug, as monotherapy carries the very real risk of encouraging the development of resistant mutants, hence the authors do not recommend it. (Immunoprophylaxis is described on p. 78.) Also there are other considerations, such as cost, side-effects and the risk of defaulting.

A final word must be said about living conditions. Poor housing and hygiene can play an important part in the spread of leprosy, and campaigns to control the disease in developing countries will have a better chance of success if they can take place on a background of improved living standards generally. The words of Latapi, the renowned Mexican leprologist, quoted by Frenken in his book,[7] are to the point:

> 'Leprosy cannot be completely rooted out with physicians, control offices, leprosaria and propaganda; it will disappear when the economic and cultural factors change, because leprosy is the thermometer of civilisation.'

REFERENCES

1 Irgens L. M. (1973). Leprosy in Norway: an interplay of research and public health work. *International Journal of Leprosy*; **41**: 189–98.

2 World Health Organization (1973). Immunological problems in leprosy research: 2. Reproduced in *Leprosy Review* (1974); **45**: 257–72.

3 Shepard C. C. (1965). Vaccination against experimental infection with *Mycobacterium leprae. American Journal of Epidemiology*; **81**: 150–63.

4 Frenken J. H. (1963). *Diffuse Leprosy of Lucio and Latapi*. Detroit, Blaine: Ethridge.

12 Differential Diagnosis

NEUROLOGICAL CONDITIONS

Palpable nerve thickening without anaesthesia or other sign of nerve damage

Excessive muscular development
This is generalised as in a professional wrestler, and localised as in a person accustomed to carry heavy weights on the head, with resultant thickening of great auricular nerve.[1]

Pachydermoperiostosis
A condition with generalised thickening of skin, periosteum and bone. Generalised nerve thickening was reported in the 3rd edition (1984) of this book. In addition there is clubbing of fingers and furrowing of the thickened skin of forehead which can easily be mistaken for the leonine facies of LL.

Palpable nerve thickening with regional anaesthesia, with or without muscle wasting

Primary amyloidosis of peripheral nerves[2]
An inherited disease which begins insidiously in second or third decades and usually affects lower limbs, with impaired sensation, muscle wasting and dropped foot. Late effects are loss of tendon reflexes and trophic ulceration of feet.

Familial hypertrophic interstitial neuritis
Déjerine–Sottas neuropathy (hereditary motor and sensory neuropathy). This begins in childhood and slowly progresses to produce muscular atrophy of limbs, commencing distally, with claw hand, dropped foot, anaesthesia, and loss of tendon reflexes.

Regional anaesthesia with or without muscle wasting but with palpable nerve thickening in some cases

Recurrent or chronic progressive (endotoxic) polyneuritis[3].
An acquired disorder of nerves – cause unknown. Symptoms first appear in adult life and tendon reflexes are diminished or absent.

Peroneal muscular atrophy (Charcot–Marie–Tooth type)
An inherited disorder, onset in childhood, with muscle weakness in lower limbs, pes cavus, hammer toes and callosities of feet. Tendon reflexes of lower limbs are diminished or absent.

Regional anaesthesia with or without muscle wasting but without palpable nerve thickening

Syringomyelia
Anaesthesia and muscle wasting develop in upper or lower limbs depending on the localisation of the cord lesion. There is dissociated anaesthesia (loss of pain and temperature sensation with preservation of touch) and tendon reflexes are diminished or lost. The histamine test is positive (see p. 65).

Tabes
Dysfunction of posterior nerve roots causes difficulty in walking due to loss of sensation and of position sense, and the patient has a broad-based stamping gait. Plantar ulceration is a later development. Eyes should be examined for Argyll–Robertson pupils, and CSF for syphilitic changes.

Peripheral neuropathy
A mononeuropathy can result from compression of nerve or nerve plexus and may simulate pure neural leprosy, e.g. cubital tunnel compression syndrome, carpal tunnel syndrome, cervical rib and meralgia paraesthetica causing sensory changes in one or both thighs. Multiple neuropathy has a large number of causes, some of which (like diabetes) result in plantar ulceration. Depression of histamine flare in anaesthetic skin is similar to that in leprosy, but there are no thickened nerves and tendon reflexes are likely to be lost.

Hereditary sensory radicular neuropathy
Loss of sensation and sweating is most severe in lower limbs, but muscular coordination is normal (compare tabes). Chronic pain-

less plantar ulceration is classical, together with high-tone deafness. Loss of ankle jerks is usual, and x-rays of feet reveal bone changes similar to those in leprosy.

Congenital indifference to pain[4]
This is seen in children who are mentally normal. Bone changes closely simulate those of leprosy, particularly absorption of terminal phalanges of fingers and tarsal bone disintegration. Histamine test is positive.

Hysteria
Caution should be observed in making this diagnosis, for the authors have treated two leprosy patients who had earlier consulted physicians in London because of regional anaesthesia and had been considered hysterical. A histamine test at that time would have been negative, thus making a diagnosis of hysteria untenable.

DERMATOLOGICAL CONDITIONS

In the conditions described in this section the reader can assume, for it will not be stated, that there is no sensory loss, there are no thickened nerves and skin smears are negative for AFB. In the few instances where this rule is broken, the deviation will be recorded. Histology is not mentioned, but it goes without stating that it is essential for diagnosis in many of these dermatoses.

Lesions which are flat and hypopigmented

1 Morphoea (localised scleroderma)
A white macule which may be slightly raised in parts, the edge often purple, hair growth and sweating are lost in the lesion, and when sclerosis is marked there is some sensory loss.

2 Onchocerciasis
A filarial infection confined to Africa, Central America and the Arabian peninsula. Depigmentation is usually confined to the pretibial regions of both legs, but may affect groins and buttocks.

3 Pityriasis alba
The circular or oval macules with fine scales are most readily noticed in children with dark skins. They are usually multiple,

principally affect the face, and tend to disappear as the child grows older.

4 Pityriasis versicolor
Readily seen in dark skins (or in sun-tanned light skins) and favouring skin covered by clothes. The macules may appear brownish. The fine branny scaling and the finding of fungal hyphae in skin scales confirm the diagnosis.

5 Post-kala-azar dermal leishmaniasis (PKDL)[5]
Although kala-azar (visceral leishmaniasis) has a very wide distribution, this late development is largely confined to the Indian subcontinent and to east Africa. Hypopigmented macules appear on trunk and limbs, rarely on face. In addition, there may be erythematous papules and nodules on face, less commonly elsewhere. There may be facial erythema with a 'butterfly' distribution over nose and cheeks. Leishman–Donovan (L–D) bodies are present in skin biopsy.

6 Yaws
A non-venereal tropical disease caused by *Treponema pertenue*. Depigmentation is a late development and is mainly confined to hairless areas of arms and tends to be bilaterally symmetrical. It occurs chiefly in adults over 30, and other signs include hyperkeratosis of palms and soles, juxta-articular nodes, gangosa, and sabre tibiae. Serological tests are positive as for syphilis.

7 Vitiligo
There is depigmentation (achromia) rather than hypopigmentation, and hairs growing in the macules may be achromic. Lesions are mutliple and of varying sizes and shapes, there are no thickened nerves and the histamine test is normal.

Lesions which are raised and pigmented

Note that in numbers 4 and 18 lesions may be flat (macular), and in number 11 they may be anaesthetic.

1 Follicular mucinosis (alopecia mucinosa)[6,7]
Cause unknown. Skin-coloured or erythematous plaques favour scalp, face, neck and shoulders. Lesions are scaly and without hairs (alopecia), but hair follicles are prominent.

2 Granuloma annulare
Cause unknown. It chiefly affects children and young adults. The typical lesion consists of erythematous or skin-coloured papules arranged in rings, and may be single or multiple. The site is commonly on extremities, and lesions run a chronic course, sometimes disappearing and later reappearing. A disseminated form is less common, consisting of papulonodules over trunk and limb.

3 Granuloma multiforme[8]
Cause unknown. This chronic dermatosis was first described in Nigeria, but has since been reported in other parts of tropical Africa. It has also been found in a region of Indonesia.[9] It chiefly affects adults over 40, and is never seen in children. Plaques closely simulate TT in appearance, but lesions irritate and sometimes new lesions appear while old ones subside.

4 Gyrate erythemas[10]
(a) *Erythema marginatum (EM)*. Macular or slightly elevated annular lesions with pink or red borders and complicating rheumatic fever, trypanosomiasis, serum sickness, or streptococcal endocarditis. (b) *Erythema chronicum migrans (ECM)*. This is the first stage of Lyme disease,[11] a spirochaetal infection resulting from the bite of a tick of the genus *Ixodes*. Within 30 days of the tick bite a small red plaque appears at the site and extends peripherally to become an erythematous annular lesion which may persist for months and attain a large size. Secondary lesions may appear at various sites, and the patients complains of headache and neck pains. (c) *Erythema gyratum repens (EGR)*. This is always associated with underlying malignant disease and presents as multiple, macular, serpiginous bands of erythema which migrate. Pruritus is common. (d) *Erythema annulare centrifugum (EAC)*. Cause is unclear, but in some cases a hypersensitivity reaction to *Tinea* infection is suspected. It usually affects young and middle-aged

adults who develop annular lesions with raised erythematous borders. These persist for weeks or months, and tend to recur over the years.

5 Kaposi's sarcoma (classical)
Aetiology not fully determined. In Africa it affects all ages and males predominantly, and presents with nodules and chronic oedema of affected limbs. Feet and lower legs are usually involved bilaterally, and legs feel hard on palpation, as in neglected LL. Oedema of legs may be the first manifestation (compare LL). Kaposi's sarcoma and AIDS is not likely to be confused with leprosy.

6 Cutaneous leishmaniasis
Early nodular lesions may simulate LL, but smears contain L–D bodies and not *M. leprae*. The type of cutaneous leishmaniasis most likely to be confused with LL is the disseminated anergic form, for nodules are numerous and simulate those of LL but are teeming with L–D bodies.

7 Lupus erythematosus
The chronic localised or discoid form usually affects women of 30–50 years of age. The round or oval plaques have a scaly surface and a predilection for face, ears and scalp. A 'butterfly' erythema of face is common. Whitish patches with red margins may appear on the buccal mucosa, and lesions on lips look like dried collodion.

8 Lupus vulgaris
Commences as a papule which coalesces with neighbouring papules to form a plaque, yellowish-red and irregular in shape. Chiefly affects the under 20s, and the face is commonly involved. The lesion becomes white when a glass slide is pressed on it, and the papules appear as brown 'apple-jelly' spots. Histological differentiation from TT is by the normal appearance of cutaneous nerves and by caseation.

9 Mycobacterium marinum *infection*
('Swimming pool' or 'fish tank' granuloma). This is a local infection of a superficial skin injury by *M. marinum*, an acid-fast mycobacterium frequenting water of swimming pools or fish tanks.

Usually a solitary erythematous nodule or plaque, sometimes becoming ulcerated and crusted. A skin smear from the lesion may contain AFB similar in appearance to *M. leprae*, but the organism can be cultured on a suitable medium. A skin test using PPD from *M. marinum* is positive.

10 Mycosis fungoides
Cause unknown, but a disorder of immunity is suspected. Presentation is with small oval or circular plaques, erythematous and finely scaling, tending to begin on buttocks and then appearing on other areas, especially trunk. These later enlarge. Lesions irritate. Occasionally there is further development into nodules which may ulcerate. Hypopigmented lesions have been reported in dark skins.

11 Necrobiosis lipoidica
Even though about 70% of patients have diabetes, the precise relationship of these two conditions is unclear. Dull red plaques appear, usually on anterior aspects of lower legs, slowly expanding and coalescing with other lesions to form annular or serpiginous lesions with central depigmentation and brown-red margins. Mann and Harman have stressed the high incidence of anaesthetic lesions.[12]

12 Atypical necrobiosis of face[13]
This occurs in adult females who are not diabetic. The annular lesions resemble borderline leprosy, but scalp is commonly involved and is diagnostic.

13 Neurofibromatosis
A congenital disorder. Nodules and oval *café au lait* (coffee-coloured) macules may well simulate LL. Nodules vary in size but are predominantly small; they also vary in colour and in consistency on palpation. Whereas the macules tend to appear in infancy, nodules usually appear at puberty. Bilateral and symmetrical nerve thickening has been reported[14] and there have been several reports of neurofibromatosis in association with leprosy.[15]

14 Pityriasis rosea
Cause unknown. Presents with many oval, rose-pink, slightly raised lesions with scaly surface and well-defined edges, character-

istically on trunk and upper half of arms and legs. Look for the 'herald patch'. Lesions disappear spontaneously in 6–10 weeks.

15 Psoriasis
A hereditary disease. Well demarcated, scaly, dull red plaques simulate scaly TT, but lesions are too numerous and involve regions such as scalp and flexures which are spared in leprosy. Fingernails may be involved.

16 Sarcoidosis[16]
Aetiology unknown. Onset is usually in the 4th to 5th decade, and every type of leprosy lesion can be mimicked by sarcoidosis, even to papules on lips, but the plaque most commonly causes confusion. Peripheral neuritis may add to this confusion, as may bone changes in hands and feet, the complication of uveitis (iridocyclitis), and the fact that skin lesions in both diseases may develop in scars.

17 Acquired syphilis[17]
The brownish-red maculopapular syphilides of secondary syphilis, and the nodulosquamous syphilides of tertiary syphilis may be confused with leprosy, especially gummatous involvement of tongue and oral mucosa with perforation of palate, but *T. pallidum* haemagglutination assay test is positive.

18 Tinea corporis (tinea circinata)
Ringworm infection of annular or plaque type may resemble leprosy, but skin scales contain the causative fungus.

19 Wegener's granulomatosis
Cause unknown, but a hypersensitivity reaction is suspected. It may be confused with LL because it usually affects young adults, begins with nasal obstruction and recurrent small epistaxes, and later develops papulonecrotic skin lesions in which vasculitis is predominant. Death frequently occurs from renal failure.

Generalised thickening of the skin

1 Systemic sclerosis (scleroderma)
Cause is incompletely understood, but genetic factors are sus-

pected. The patient develops a taut and thickened skin which slowly becomes bound to subcutaneous tissues, recurrent ulcerations develop at the ends of fingers, and terminal phalanges become absorbed. Polyarthritis of small joints is common, and finger contractures may develop.

2 Myxoedema
A condition due to thyroid underactivity. It has many similarities to LL – thickening of skin, thinning of eyebrows, a hoarse voice, oedematous legs, a normocytic normochromic anaemia, and carpal tunnel syndrome as a complication.

3 Pachydermoperiostosis
A familial condition predominantly affecting males, in which the facial appearance, with deepening of the lines of face and forehead, closely resembles LL. Bone changes take the form of proliferative periostitis, fingers become thickened, and there is clubbing of fingers and toes.

REFERENCES

1 Dharmendra (1980). Thickened nerves in diagnosis of leprosy. *Leprosy in India*; **52**: 1–2.
2 Andrade C. (1953). A peculiar form of peripheral neuropathy. Familiar atypical generalized amyloidosis with special involvement of peripheral nerves. *Brain*; **75**: 408–27.
3 Harris W. (1935). Chronic progressive (endotoxic) polyneuritis. *Brain*; **58**: 368–75.
4 Sandell L. J. (1958). Congenital indifference to pain. *Journal of the Faculty of Radiologists*; **9**: 50–6.
5 Munro D. D., du Vivier A., Jopling W. H. (1972). Post-kala azar dermal leishmaniasis. *British Journal of Dermatology*; **87**: 374–8.
6 Pinkus H. (1957). Alopecia mucinosa. *Archives of Dermatology*; **76**: 419–26.
7 Fan J., Chang H., Ma B. (1967). Alopecia mucinosa simulating leprosy. *Archives of Dermatology*; **95**: 354–6.
8 Leiker D. L., Kok S. H., Spaas J. A. J. (1964). Granuloma multiforme: a new disease resembling leprosy. *International Journal of Leprosy*; **32**: 368–76.

9 Leiker D. L. (1971). Distribution of granuloma multiforme. *International Journal of Leprosy*; **39**: 189.
10 Willis W. F. (1978). The gyrate erythemas. *International Journal of Dermatology*; **17**: 698–702.
11 Habicht G. S., Beck G., Benach J. L. (1987). Lyme Disease. *Scientific American*; **257**: 60–5.
12 Mann R. J., Harman R. R. M. (1984). Cutanous anaesthesia in necrobiosis lipoidica. *British Journal of Dermatology*; **110**: 323–5.
13 Dowling G. B., Wilson Jones E. (1967). Atypical (annular) necrobiosis lipoidica of the face and scalp. *Dermatologica*; **135**: 11–26.
14 Naik R. P. C., Srinivas C. R., Rao R. V. (1985). Thickening of nerves in neurofibromatosis. *Indian Journal of Leprosy*; **57**: 876–8.
15 Joseph M. S. (1985). Von Recklinghausen's disease associated with diffuse lepromatous leprosy. *Indian Journal of Leprosy*; **57**: 872–5.
16 James D. G., Jopling W. H. (1961). Sarcoidosis and leprosy. *Journal of Tropical Medicine and Hygiene*; **64**: 42–6.
17 Nsibambi J. K. (1981). Leprosy and syphilis: a case report. *Leprosy Review*; **52**: 171–3.

Glossary

Abduction (of fingers). The act of separating them.

Acedapsone. An acetyl derivative of dapsone suitable for intramuscular injection every 3 months. Also known as DADDS and Hansolar.

Adduction (of fingers). The act of approximating them.

Aetiology. The cause or origin of a disease.

Agranulocytosis. Complete or nearly complete absence of granulocytes from the blood, i.e. the polymorphonuclears, eosinophils and basophils.

AIDS (Acquired immunodeficiency syndrome). A chronic disease caused by the human immunodeficiency virus (HIV) in which cell-mediated immunity is depressed. It can be transmitted by blood, semen and cervical secretions. A virus with west African connections is named HIV–II.

Allograft. A portion of tissue removed from a donor to be applied to a recipient of the same species, e.g. from one human to another.

Alopecia. Deficiency of hair.

Alveolar (maxillary). Pertaining to the tooth socket.

Amblyopia. Dimness of vision.

Amyloidosis. The formation of amyloid (starchy) substance in various tissues. The term 'secondary amyloidosis' implies a complication of chronic sepsis or of certain chronic diseases.

Anhidrosis. Deficiency or absence of the secretion of sweat.

Ankylosis. Abnormal immobility of a joint.

Annular. Shaped like a ring.

Anorexia. Loss of appetite for food.

Anosmia. Loss of the sense of smell.

Antibody. A substance in the body which reacts with a specific antigen.

Antigen. A substance which when introduced into the body causes the formation of antibody.

Aqueous humour. The fluid filling the anterior chamber of the eye.

Arachis oil. Peanut (groundnut) oil.

Argyll–Robertson pupils. Pupils which react to accommodation but not to light.

Arthrodesis. The surgical fixation of a joint.

Arthus reaction. An inflammatory reaction to the presence of antigen in a human or animal that has already been sensitised to that antigen; antigen–antibody complexes, in the presence of complement, adhere to the endothelium of small blood vessels, become surrounded by fibrin, platelets and neutrophils, resulting in thrombosis, tissue necrosis, and exudation of fluid and blood from the damaged vessels into surrounding tissues.

Autonomic nerve. A nerve belonging to a system of nerves acting independently of the will and not controlled by the will, e.g. the nerves controlling blood vessels, cardiac action and peristalsis.

Axon (axis cylinder). A tiny nerve fibre conducting impulses.

Azoospermia. Absence of spermatozoa in the semen.

Bactericidal. Having a direct antibacterial effect. Therefore killing bacteria quickly.

Bacteriostatic. Having an indirect antibacterial effect, e.g. by interfering with bacterial nutrition. Therefore killing bacteria slowly.

BCG vaccine. A vaccine made from bacillus Calmette-Guérin, an avirulent strain of bovine tubercle bacilli.

BI. Bacterial Index, i.e. the concentration of bacilli in a skin smear or biopsy.

Bell's palsy. Facial paralysis of acute onset due to inflammation of the facial nerve within the stylomastoid foramen.

Biopsy. Removal of a piece of tissue from a living subject for diagnostic purposes.

Biopsy index. A method of showing both the bacterial density and the size of a skin lesion.

Bulla. A rounded bleb or blister formed by the accumulation of fluid within or beneath the epidermis. It differs from a vesicle only in its larger size and in the fact that it does not occur in groups.

Calcification. The process by which a tissue becomes hardened by deposition of calcium salts within it.

Callosity. A circumscribed thickening and hardening of the skin.

Capillary. One of the microscopic blood vessels forming a network connecting arterioles and venules.

Carpal tunnel syndrome. Pain in the palm from compression of median nerve in the wrist.

Carville. The official United States hospital for the treatment of leprosy. It is situated in Louisiana.

Cataract (ocular). A hard opacity situated within the lens or beneath the capsule of the lens.

Chaulmoogra oil. An oil obtained from the seeds of a tree indigenous to southern Asia, formerly used in the treatment of leprosy.

Cell-mediated immunity (CMI). Specific immunity that is mediated by small lymphocytes which are thymus-dependent and known as T cells or T lymphocytes.

Cellulitis. Purulent inflammation of subcutaneous tissue.

Chondrocyte. A mature cartilage cell.

Ciliary body. Situated in the anterior part of the eye on either side of the lens, the two ciliary bodies play an important part in accommodation, i.e. in altering the shape of the lens when looking at near objects. Together with the iris and choroid it forms the uvea (or uveal tract), the coloured layer of the eye.

Claw fingers (claw hand). The affected fingers are extended (dorsiflexed) at the metacarpophalangeal joint and flexed at the first interphalangeal joint.

Cold abscess. An abscess of slow development with little evidence of inflammation.

Collagen. A substance which is found in the walls of all blood vessels; it is a safety factor for the vessel, preventing it 'blowing out' at high pressure.

Complement. A system of serologically non-specific proteins present in serum that are necessary for the lysis or death of antigens in the presence of antibody.

Concentric. Having a common centre. The term 'concentric bone absorption' signifies an equal loss of bone in all directions from a common centre.

Conjunctivitis. Inflammation of the conjunctiva (the delicate membrane lining the eyelids and covering the eye in front).

Cornea. The transparent structure forming the anterior part of the external layer of the eyeball.

Corneal microscope. A powerful microscope for direct examination of the anterior structures of the eye, particularly the cornea and iris, with the patient seated in front of the examiner.

Corticosteroid. A hormone produced by the adrenal cortex (cortisol) or a related synthetic hormone of greater activity weight for weight (prednisone; prednisolone; triamcinolone; dexamethasone, etc.).

CSF. Cerebrospinal fluid.

Cubital tunnel syndrome. Pain in the elbow from compression of ulnar nerve at that point.

Cushing's disease. A disease due to overgrowth or to an adenoma of the basophil cells of the anterior lobe of the pituitary gland.

Cushing's syndrome. Symptoms and signs suggestive of Cushing's disease and due to prolonged treatment with large doses of corticosteroid.

Cutaneous. Pertaining to the skin.

Cyanosis. A blue colour of the skin which occurs when there is more than 5 g of reduced haemoglobin per 100 ml of blood in the capillaries.

Cyclitis. Inflammation of the ciliary body. The term 'plastic cyclitis' implies cyclitis with exudation of fibrinous matter into the anterior chamber of the eye.

Dactylitis. Inflammation of one or more fingers or toes.

DADDS. See **Acedapsone.**

Danielssen. Daniel Cornelius, 1815–1894, Norwegian dermatologist.

Demyelination. Loss of the myelin of nerve tissue, whether affecting brain, spinal cord, or peripheral nerve.

Depigmentation. Complete loss of pigment.

Dermis. The true skin (also known as cutis or corium) lying between the epidermis and the subcutaneous tissue.

Desquamate. To shed the surface of the skin (epidermis) in scales or sheets.

Diasone sodium. Sodium sulfoxone. A di-substituted sulphone which breaks down to produce small quantities of dapsone after hydrolysis in the stomach. It is an expensive form of administering dapsone and has largely been abandoned in the treatment of leprosy.

Dimorphous. Having two forms.

DNA. Deoxyribonucleic acid.

Dorsal surface. See **Extensor surface.**

Dorsum. The back of the body or of a limb, or the side on which the extensor muscles function.

Electron microscope. A microscope in which a beam of electron waves is used, giving much greater magnification than that of an ordinary microscope using a beam of light waves (a light microscope).

Endarteritis. Inflammation of the inner lining of arteries or arterioles.

Endemic disease. One which is prevalent in a particular region.

Endogenous. Having origin within the organism.

Endoneurium. Within a nerve, the sheath of fine connective tissue surrounding each nerve fibre.

Enteric coating. A coating given to a tablet to ensure that it will pass unchanged through the stomach and duodenum into the jejunum.

Epidemiological curve (of tuberculosis). If the incidence of tuberculosis in any given country is studied over a period of a hundred or more years from the time of its introduction to that country, it will show a steady increase, will reach a maximum, and then will slowly decrease as successive generations in that population acquire genetic immunity.

Epidermis. The outermost, and non-vascular, layer of the skin.

Epididymis. An oblong body attached to the upper part of each testis (testicle).

Epididymo-orchitis. Inflammation of epididymis and testis (testicle).

Epineurium. The sheath of connective tissue surrounding a nerve trunk.

Epistaxis. Nose bleeding.

Epithelioid cell. A fixed macrophage cell which is characteristically found in certain chronic infections such as tuberculosis and leprosy. Its presence in the tissues is evidence that the host possesses cell-mediated immunity; hence it is found in the tuberculoid type of leprosy but not in the lepromatous type.

Epitope. A small molecular region within an antigen which activates T and B lymphocytes (T and B cells).

Erysipelas. An acute disease of the skin due to haemolytic streptococci and characterised by fever, constitutional symptoms, and bright red patches on the skin.

Escherichia coli. Commonly spoken of as *Bacillus coli (B. coli)*. It is a short Gram-negative motile bacillus which is a normal inhabitant of the large bowel, but in certain other organs it acts as a pathogen, e.g. urinary tract and biliary tract.

ESR. Erythrocyte sedimentation rate.

Etiology. See Aetiology.

Extensor surface. The surface of a limb which covers the extensor muscles (the muscles which extend the joints).

Fasciculus. A bundle of nerve fibres. Alternative names are nerve bundle and funiculus.

Fastigium. The highest point of a fever.

Fibrosis. The formation of fibrous tissue.

Fixative. A fluid in which to place a biopsy prior to sectioning and staining.

Flexor surface. The surface of a limb which covers the flexor muscles (the muscles which flex the joints).

Fluctuant. When applied to a swelling it means that finger pressure at one side of the swelling can be felt by a finger at the opposite side, and this implies that the swelling contains fluid.

Foam cell. When biopsy sections stained with H & E are examined with a microscope, macrophages have a foamy appearance (and are called foam cells) if they contain a high proportion of dead leprosy bacilli. The foamy appearance is due to fat.

Funiculus. See **Fasciculus.**

Generation time (of a bacterium). The time taken to divide into two (binary fission).

Genetic. Pertaining to genes – inherited.

Giant cell (of Langhans). A large multinucleated cell resembling a horse-shoe in shape and formed by epithelioid cells grouping together. It is characteristic of certain chronic infections, such as tuberculosis and leprosy (tuberculoid type).

Glaucoma. A painful condition in which the intra-ocular pressure is raised.

Globus. A lepra cell seen in a section or smear after suitable staining.

Granulocyte. A cell containing granules, especially a leucocyte (white blood cell) containing neutrophil, basophil or eosinophil granules in its cytoplasm, i.e. a polymorphonuclear, basophil or eosinophil cell.

Granuloma. In a section of a leprosy lesion examined under the microscope the granuloma is the collection of defensive cells (the cellular reaction), particularly when cell-mediated immunity is present.

H. & E. Haematoxylin and Eosin stain.

Haematemesis (hematemesis). The act of vomiting blood.

Haemolytic (hemolytic) anaemia. Anaemia due to disruption of red blood cells and loss of haemoglobin from the cells into the plasma.

Half-life. The time taken, from the time of ingesting a drug, for its concentration in the blood to be reduced to 50% of its original value.

Hammer toe. A condition in which the proximal (first) phalanx is extended (dorsiflexed) and the second phalanx is flexed. The claw finger is its counterpart in the hand.

Hansen. Gerhard Henrik Armauer, 1841–1912, Norwegian leprologist.

Hansolar. See **Acedapsone.**

Hepatitis. Inflammation of the liver.

Histiocyte. A mononuclear phagocytic cell of the tissues derived from the monocytes (large mononuclears) of the blood, forming part of the reticuloendothelial system. A characteristic cell in lepromatous leprosy. See **Macrophage.**

Histoid. Web-like. 'Histoid leproma' is a term introduced by Wade to describe the histological appearance of hyperactive lepromatous nodules sometimes seen in relapsed cases or in patients whose bacilli have become resistant to treatment.

HLA. Human leucocyte antigen.

Humoral immunity. Immunity pertaining to body fluids, in contrast with cellular (cell-mediated) immunity. It is initiated by small lymphocytes which are thymus-independent and known as

B cells or B lymphocytes; these differentiate into plasma cells secreting immunoglobulins.

Hyalase. Trade name for hyaluronidase.

Hyaluronidase. An enzyme known as the 'spreading factor'. When injected with fluid into the skin or subcutaneous tissue it facilitates the spread of the fluid through the intercellular spaces.

Hyperpigmentation. Increased pigment or colouring.

Hypertension. Raised blood pressure.

Hypochromia. See **Hypopigmentation.**

Hypopigmentation. Reduced pigment or colouring.

Hypothenar. Pertaining to the ulnar (median) margin of the palm.

Ichthyosis. Skin having a dry, fish-scale appearance.

ILEP. International Federation of Antileprosy Associations.

IMMLEP. Immunology of leprosy. A research programme under the aegis of WHO.

Impotence. Inability to perform the sex act.

Incidence. The number of new cases of a particular disease which occur in a defined population during a specific period of time. The time period used is conventionally 1 year, but it may be longer, e.g. 5 years.

Incisor. The incisor teeth are the four front teeth of either jaw.

Institutionalisation. Loss of will to be independent and to fend for oneself resulting from long-continued stay in an institution such as a hospital.

Insomnia. Inability to sleep.

Intrinsic. Situated entirely within a part, e.g. intrinsic muscles of the hand begin and end in the hand.

***In vitro*.** Outside the body.

***In vivo*.** Within the body.

Iridectomy. Surgical removal of part of the iris.

Iridocyclitis. Inflammation of iris and ciliary body.

Iris. The circular coloured membrane behind the cornea and perforated by the pupil. Together with the ciliary body and the choroid it forms the uvea (uveal tract) – the coloured layer of the eye.

Iris bombé. Umbrella iris. A condition in which the iris is bowed forward by the collection of aqueous humour between the iris and the lens in total posterior synechia, i.e. when the iris is bound to the pupil posteriorly.

Iritis. Inflammation of the iris.

Irradiation. In medical treatment this usually applies to radiotherapy – treatment with x-rays or other form of radioactivity.

Keratitis. Inflammation of the cornea.

Lagophthalmos. Inability to approximate the eyelids.

Langhans cells. See **Giant Cell.**

Lazar hospital. Medieval term for leprosy hospital or leprosarium.

Leonine. Lion-like.

LEPRA. British Leprosy Relief Association, Fairfax House, Causton Road, Colchester, Essex CO1 1PU.

Lepra cell. A wandering macrophage cell packed full of leprosy bacilli.

Leproma. A nodule of lepromatous leprosy. The term, as used by histologists, signifies the cellular reaction in lepromatous leprosy.

Leprosarium. A hospital or colony for the isolation and treatment of leprosy patients.

Leucoderma (leukoderma). Skin depigmentation from any cause.

Lymphadenitis. Inflammation of lymph glands.

Lymphadenopathy. Enlargement of lymph glands.

Lymphoedema (lymphedema). Swelling due to back pressure of lymph when lymph flow is impaired.

Lymphokines. Substances released by T lymphocytes when they come into contact with antigen to which they have become sensitised.

Macrophage. A histiocyte which has engulfed leprosy bacilli and either forms a wandering macrophage or lepra cell (in LL) or a fixed epithelioid cell (in TT).

Macule. A skin lesion which is not elevated above the surface of the skin and therefore cannot be felt by the examining finger.

Madarosis. Loss of eyelashes (ciliary madarosis) or of eyebrows (superciliary madarosis).

***Main de Singe*.** Ape Hand. A hand with wasting of thenar muscles and paralysis of thumb due to median nerve damage.

Main de griffe. See **Claw fingers.**

Manic-depressive. A form of psychosis in which the mood tends to alternate between elevation and depression.

Maxillary. Pertaining to the maxilla or upper jaw.

Melanocyte. Any pigment-bearing cell such as that found in the skin, or in the choroid coat of the eyeball.

Metacarpal. One of the five cylindrical bones of the hand connecting the carpus (wrist) with the fingers.

Metatarsal. One of the five bones of the foot connecting the tarsus with the toes.

Metatarsectomy. Surgical removal of the whole of, or a part of, a metatarsal bone.

Methaemoglobinaemia (methemoglobinemia). A modified form of oxyhaemoglobin found in the blood after ingestion of certain drugs and sometimes giving the lips and skin a blue colour.

MI. Morphological Index. The percentage of solid-staining bacilli in a smear or biopsy.

Miliary. Characterised by the formation of lesions resembling millet seeds.

Miosis. Abnormal contraction of the pupil.

Mitogen. A substance which stimulates mitosis (cell division), e.g. phytohaemagglutinin derived from kidney bean.

Monoclonal antibody. Derived from a single clone of B lymphocytes (B cells).

Mononeuritic. Affecting only one nerve.

Mononeuritis. Inflammation of one nerve.

Monotherapy. Treatment with one drug.

Morbidity. The condition of being diseased.

Morphology. Structure.

Mucosa. The lining or mucous membrane of parts of the body in contact with air, e.g. mouth, pharynx, trachea, bronchi, gastrointestinal tract.

Multibacillary. Moderate or large numbers of bacilli.

Mutant. In leprosy the word signifies a strain of bacilli resistant to the drug in use.

Myxoedema (myxedema). A disease due to reduced function of the thyroid gland.

Nausea. Desire to vomit.

Necrosis. Death of a circumscribed portion of tissue.

Neelsen. Friederich Karl Adolf, 1854–1894, German bacteriologist.

Neonatal. Referring to the newborn.

Nephritis. Inflammation of the kidney.

Neurolysis. Nerve decompression. The surgical relief of pressure within a nerve, and involves either incising or stripping the nerve sheath.

Nocturnal. Pertaining to the night.

Nodule. A tumour or protuberance of the skin measuring more than 10 mm in diameter.

Nomenclature. Terminology.

Normochromic. Normal in colour.

Normocytic. Normal in size.

Osteoblast. One of the cells directly active in the production of bone.

Osteomyelitis. Infection of bone.

Osteoporosis. A condition of bones in which they become more porous (less dense) and therefore less strong. Also known as rarefaction.

Pannus. A network of dilated superficial blood vessels in the cornea associated with a cellular infiltration.

Papule. A small protuberance of the skin less than 10 mm in diameter.

Paraesthesia (paresthesia). Abnormal sensation.

Parenteral. Not through the alimentary canal, i.e. either subcutaneous, intramuscular or intravenous.

Pathogen. Any disease-producing micro-organism or material.

Pathognomonic. Indicative of a particular disease.

Paucillary. Few bacilli or none.

Peptic ulceration. Ulceration of stomach or duodenum.

Perineurium. Within a nerve, the sheath of fine connective tissue surrounding each bundle of nerve fibres.

Periostitis. Inflammation of the periosteum (the fibrous membrane surrounding a bone).

Phagocyte. A cell capable of ingesting, and usually digesting, various substances, particularly micro-organisms.

Phalanx. One of the bones of finger or toe.

Phthisis bulbi. A soft, shrunken, blind eye.

PHA. Phytohaemagglutination.

Pituitary. The ductless gland situated in the pituitary fossa of the sphenoid bone the anterior part of which secretes hormones which stimulate various organs, e.g. adrenocorticotrophic hormone (ACTH) which stimulates the adrenal cortex to produce cortisol. The pituitary gland is also known as the hypophysis cerebri.

Plantar. Pertaining to the sole of the foot.

Plantaris tendon. The long slender tendon of plantaris muscle travelling down the back of the leg to be inserted into the posterior part of the calcaneum.

Plasma. The fluid (non-cellular) portion of the blood before clotting has occurred.

Plastazote. Polyethylene foam splinting material used for various orthopaedic purposes. In leprosy its particular use is in the form of insoles for shoes or lining of sandals, as it can be moulded so as to relieve pressure on prominences. Shoes or boots can be made entirely of Plastazote. Technical information is obtainable from Smith & Nephew Ltd, Bessemer Road, Welwyn Garden City, Hertfordshire, England.

Plaque. A disc-shaped skin lesion which can be felt by the examining finger. Sometimes it is formed by the extension or coalescence of papules or nodules.

Polyclonal antibody. Derived from multiple clones of B lymphocytes (B cells).

Polymorphs. Polymorphonuclear cells or neutrophil granulocytes. Multinucleated white blood cells derived from myelocytes in the red marrow and composing roughly 60% of the white cells in health.

Polyneuritic. Affecting several (or many) nerves.

Prednisone. A drug used similarly to cortisone but given in one-fifth the dose. It causes less electrolyte disturbance than cortisone, i.e. less retention of sodium and less elimination of potassium.

Prevalence. The number of cases of a particular disease in a defined population at a specific time.

Prevalence rate. The number of cases of a particular disease at a specific time, divided by the population in which these cases occur.

Prognosis. Outlook for cure.

Promin. Sodium glucosulphone. The first sulphone used in leprosy but now largely abandoned as it has to be administered intravenously.

Proteinuria. Protein in the urine.

Psychosis. A disease or disorder of the mind.

Ptyalism. A condition in which there is increased flow of saliva.

Pumice (pumice stone). A very light porous stone of volcanic origin and grey in colour.

Punctate. Marked with points or dots.

Pupil (of eye). The opening at the centre of the iris for the transmission of light and for controlling the quantity of light transmitted by means of dilatation or contraction.

Purpura. Red or purple patches in the skin or mucous membrane caused by extravasation of blood. The colour does not disappear on pressure by the examining finger.

Pustule. A small well-defined elevation of the skin containing pus.

Pyelonephritis. Inflammation of the kidney and its pelvis.

Rhinitis. Inflammation of the mucous membrane of the nose.

RNA. Ribonucleic acid.

Round cell. Another word for lymphocyte (a variety of white blood corpuscle) and usually used to describe lymphocytes deposited in the skin as a defensive reaction.

Schick needle. A fine hypodermic needle 1·3 cm long.

Schizoid. Resembling schizophrenia, i.e. the shut-in, dreamy, unsocial, lonely type of person.

Sclera. The tough white coat surrounding the eyeball excepting for the anterior segment covered by the cornea. It is the 'white' of the eye.

Scleritis. Inflammation of the sclera.

Scleroderma. A disease in which a diffuse thickening of the skin is the cardinal sign.

Sclerosing. Hardening as a result of inflammation.

Sclerotic. Pertaining to the sclera.

Schwann cell. A phagocytic cell attached to a peripheral nerve fibre.

Sebaceous. Pertaining to sebum (the greasy secretion of the skin).

Segregation. Separation from others.

Serpiginous. Creeping from one part or surface to another.

Serum. Blood serum is the clear liquid which separates from the blood after clotting.

Shelf-life (of a drug). The time between date of manufacture and date of expiry.

Spindle-shape. Thickened in the middle and tapering at both ends.

Steroid. See **Coricosteroid.**

Stigma. A mark of infamy or disgrace.

Stridor. A loud and harsh sound produced by breathing when there is airway obstruction.

Sulphetrone. The proprietary name for solapsone – a di-substituted sulphone suitable for oral or parenteral administration in the treatment of leprosy, but now no longer marketed.

Syme's amputation. Amputation of the foot at the ankle joint with removal of both malleoli.

Synechia. Adhesion. In ophthalmology, an adhesion formed between the iris and the cornea, or the lens, following an attack of iritis or iridocyclitis.

Synergism. The enhanced antibacterial effect when two drugs are used concurrently.

Systemic. Affecting the body as a whole

Taelangiectasis (telangiectasis). Dilatation of capillary vessels and minute arterioles in the skin.

TALMILEP. A committee within ILEP (see p. 138) devoted to teaching and learning materials on the subject of leprosy.

Tarsorrhaphy. The operation of suturing together the upper and lower eyelids, either entirely (total tarsorrhaphy) or partially (partial tarsorrhaphy).

Testis. Testicle. The male gonad.

Testosterone. The male hormone produced by the testis.

THELEP. Chemotherapy of Leprosy. A research programme under the aegis of WHO.

Thenar. The region of the palm at the base of the thumb. The principal thenar muscles are the opponens pollicis and the abductor pollicis brevis, both supplied by the median nerve.

Thioamide. The name of a group of medicinal substances which includes ethionamide and prothionamide.

Thrombocytosis. Increase in the number of thrombocytes (platelets).

Thymectomy. Surgical removal of the thymus.

Thymus. A gland situated behind the sternum (breast bone) and concerned with the development of immunity. The 'primary' lymphoid organ. It involutes after puberty.

Tracheotomy. The surgical establishment of an opening into the trachea through the anterior aspect of the neck.

Tranquilliser. A drug which relieves nervous tension without imparing consciousness.

Trauma. Injury.

Trimester. A period of three months.

Triple arthrodesis. Surgical fusion of the following joints of the foot: (1) subtalar; (2) calcaneocuboid; (3) talonavicular.

Tuberculoid. Resembling tuberculosis. Histologically this means the presence of lymphocytes, epithelioid cells and Langhans giant cells.

Ulcer. An open sore other than a wound.

Vasculitis. Inflammation of the inner lining of blood vessels.

Vertigo. Dizziness; giddiness.

Vesicle. A small rounded bleb or blister formed by the accumulation of fluid within or beneath the epidermis. Vesicles often occur in groups.

Vesicular. Pertaining to or made up of vesicles on the skin.

Vitiligo. A skin disease of unknown aetiology characterised by white (depigmented) macules, due to destruction of pigment cells of the epidermis. Sometimes the hairs within the macules become white.

Vitreous body. The transparent substance of the consistency of thin jelly, enclosed within the hyaloid membrane, which occupies about four-fifths of the eyeball.

Xanthelasma palpebrarum. Soft yellow spots or plaques seen in the regions of the eyelids in a small proportion of persons above middle age. Although the patients are usually healthy, the condition may be associated with diabetes, arteriosclerosis, lepromatous leprosy, xanthoma tuberosum or xanthoma disseminatum.

Yaws. A treponemal disease of the tropics, acquired non-venereally, and chiefly affecting the skin.

Ziehl. Franz Ziehl, 1857–1926, German bacteriologist.

Zoonosis. A disease common to man and other animals, usually in which animals are the main reservoir of infection.

Zygomatic. Pertaining to the zygoma, the malar bone (cheek bone).

Index